Thyroid Adrenal
Secrets Revealed!

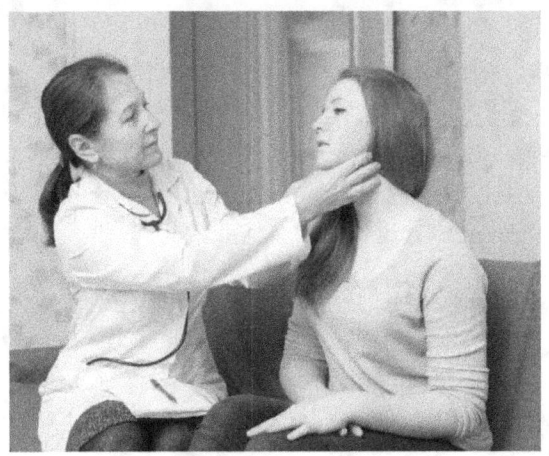

A Thyroid Adrenal Guide

Attention: If you seek answers before visiting your doctor or just a natural approach to thyroid and adrenal health, you have found it. This book contains secrets all people should know. Check it out – you may find a tip or two that could change your life for the better!

Other Books by ABC Wellness in the "Simple Steps to Better Health" Series:

Calming Inflammation: The eBook "Autoimmune and Inflammation Solutions" gives you a Natural Recovery Protocol to Overcome Food Allergies, Gluten, GMOs, EMFs, Biofilms, Yeast or Candida Overgrowth. Only 99 cents!

Dental and Heart Care: The eBook, "Reversing Gum And Heart Disease" provides a Protocol to Lower hs-CRP, and Heal Inflammation Through a Paleo Diet, Dental Care, and Targeted Nutrients and Supplements. Only $2.99!

Thyroid and Adrenal Facts: The eBook "Thyroid Adrenal Secrets Revealed" teaches you what you the 10 top things you need to know before you see your doctor for thyroid or adrenal issues.

Analyze and Improve Your Health: The eBook "25 Step Healing Program" gives you simple steps to take to evaluate your health and improve it by correcting deficiencies.

Improve Your Health Safely: The eBook "Heal Your Whole Body Naturally" covers using bio identical hormones as well as a natural approach to staying well.

Lose Pounds Quickly by Overcoming Obstacles to Weightloss: The eBook "The ABC Wellness

Weightloss Pyramid" covers 9 major obstacles or possible roadblocks that once removed will help you lose weight without dieting or exercise, though that is recommended to compound your gains.

Acid Reflux or GERD: The eBook "Acid Reflux Relief Now" allows you to stop heartburn or acid reflux in its tracks with natural remedies.

Anti-Aging Secrets: The eBook "Insider Bio Identical Hormone Secrets and More" covers the secrets you need to know to stay young and health with the use of natural hormones.

Longevity and Anti-Aging Advice: The eBook "How to Live to 100 – Top Dos and Don'ts" gives you the top 10 dos and don'ts you should follow if you want to reach and surpass the golden age of 100.

Thyroid, Adrenals and Weightloss: The eBook "Thyroid Adrenal Weightloss Solutions" covers the 25 steps in the "25 Step Healing Program" book, along with more information on losing pounds quickly.

Special note on Thyroid Adrenal Weightloss Solutions: This is a modified version of the "25 Step Healing Program" eBook, so please purchase this one if you want more information on losing weight as well as the thyroid, adrenal and testing information.

Please forgive us if any sites referenced in our eBooks are not operational when you visit them, and please try back later, as they may be under construction. Thank-you!

SPECIAL ANNOUNCEMENTS

To see a free video on thyroid adrenal care and for an even more comprehensive video based program, and for free gifts and articles on thyroid and adrenals by email, please visit and sign up at http://thyroid-adrenal-solutions.com

Thyroid Adrenal
Secrets Revealed!

10 Things to Know before You See Your Doctor for Thyroid Disease including Lab Tests, Physical Exams Findings, Symptoms, Toxic Exposures, Supplements, Adrenal Evaluation, Food Allergy Evaluation, and Natural Hormone Treatment

Diane Culik, MD
Kyle Weed, Editor

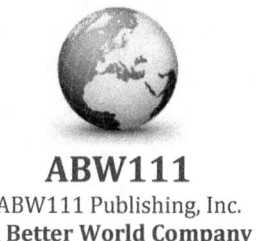

ABW111
ABW111 Publishing, Inc.
A Better World Company

Thyroid Adrenal Secrets Revealed

Thyroid Adrenal
Secrets Revealed!

This book is dedicated to those individuals who seek answers for their thyroid and adrenal questions either for self-enlightenment or before they visit their doctor. It gives natural solutions and secrets that can lift one from despair to on the road to recovery.

"Natural forces within us are the true healers of disease." ~Hippocrates

"I saw a woman wearing a sweatshirt with 'Guess' on it. I said, 'Thyroid Problem?'" ~Arnold Schwarzenegger

"I want people to know that blood tests alone won't always detect thyroid disease. My blood panels were normal. I think a lot more people have this disease than are diagnosed." ~Kim Alexis

TABLE OF CONTENTS

INTRODUCTION

WHAT IS THIS BOOK ABOUT?

Do you remember how it felt to just feel great? Think back to when life was easy, you were younger, and things looked bright indeed. Wouldn't it be nice to feel that way again? We feel this may be possible – that there are certain factors playing a role in not feeling so well for millions of people. One of these things is the foods and nutrition we consume, and another is the toxins that are affecting all of us today. But we look at much more than just that – stay with us and we will help you find some answers that perhaps no one has been able to give you so far.

This book reveals valuable information about the thyroid and adrenal glands – how to properly test for problems with these glands, how to interpret test results, what physical exam findings might reveal, what symptoms are exhibited when problems exist, and what toxins play a role in their functioning and need to be avoided.

Next, it covers what supplements will help you feel better, how food allergies play a part, and why natural thyroid hormone is best if you need it. Much more follows and some timeless secrets are revealed. Discover what you need to know to recognize thyroid and adrenal problems and properly treat these glands so you feel great again!

Why write a book about the thyroid and adrenals?

Everyone has these glands, and far too people are not feeling as good as they might. In fact, it is estimated that 60 million or more people suffer from some type of thyroid disorder, and most people don't even recognize it. In our toxic, often stress filled world, many more suffer from adrenal dysfunction, and the thyroid and adrenal glands affect each other's functioning. So they should be evaluated together as part of the whole body's system, and each person should be treated with a holistic, safe, natural approach that addresses the problem at the causative level, not just symptomatically.

On top of all this, there is a lot of misinformation out there, so our goal is to quickly get you the information you need so your thyroid and adrenals are properly tested and treated, and to give you actionable things you can do right now to feel your best. This book will give you safe tips to help your thyroid and adrenal glands function, and perhaps just as importantly, prepare you to talk to your doctor so that you are properly evaluated and treated.

About the Authors - who are we and why should you listen to us?

This book is a collaboration between Diane Culik, MD, and Kyle Weed, independent health researcher. When two people work together, the end result of their efforts is often synergistic, and much more benefit is derived by the end consumer. What follows below is a write-up for each of us, and then a short explanation as to why we working together will benefit you as someone wishing to improve their health.

Dr. Diane Culik, MD, brings you natural health solutions, and is a top thyroid-adrenal doctor with over 30 years' experience! After graduating from the University of Michigan Medical School, Dr. Culik began practicing medicine a number of years ago, following the traditional path, learning the best that conventional medicine had to offer.

About 17 years ago, she switched to Holistic Medicine, and now blends the two approaches so you get the best of both worlds! She recently opened ABC Wellness, which stands for Alternative-Balanced-Comprehensive, in Sterling Heights, Michigan where she offers all patients "Simple Steps to Better Health." Her goal is to assist you in finding the path to a better way of life through the removal of obstacles to healing like environmental toxins and nutritional deficiencies and allowing the body to heal itself.

Kyle Weed is an independent health researcher, a writer, and communicator, with a "Vision" of reaching people through a variety of media and creating happiness, healing, and peace. He currently works with ABC Wellness to create eBooks, and DVD/Video Programs on Natural Health Topics such as anti-aging, cancer survival secrets, thyroid and adrenal care, weightloss, and more.

Kyle felt led to this experience through inner guidance after years of suffering through mercury toxicity caused in part by "silver" fillings, and after extensively researching the health field, reading through hundreds of health and medical books, websites and other literature. His goal is to bring Alternative Health Secrets, both ancient and new and unique Healing Modalities, Forgiveness and Mind Training Techniques and any other helpful healing information to public awareness.

How do the two of us working together offer a greater benefit to you, the reader, and user of possible life changing alternative health secrets?

By working together, the two of us fill in gaps each one of us working and writing independently may have missed. Dr. Culik provides the credibility of a trained medical doctor, can offer authoritative knowledge on many topics, and also the safety factor only a trained medical professional can offer, while still retaining a mind open to new and unusual alternative healing techniques.

She will be the one providing the step by step instructions for this eBook based on her experience with patients, and her knowledge of thyroid and adrenal issues.

Kyle Weed, having undergone a lengthy health challenge and an equally lengthy period of studying health techniques and information can often definitively state in many cases what really worked to bring healing and comfort to himself and others undergoing similar experiences.

As I (Kyle Weed) am the one pulling the information together, and adding to it, I can state that I have personally read and studied tons of material from the leading alternative, natural doctors on the scene today, so both Dr. Culik and I will bring you the best of the best in alternative health care, including top secrets you can use right now!

Disclaimer: Of course, we have to state that this information is for educational purposes only, and not meant to substitute for medical attention. If you have concerns with anything you want to try as a result of your learning here, please see your primary physician. Most things we mention are proven to be safe - foods, supplements, and testing methods you can try at home inexpensively, but please do err on the side of caution when trying anything. Start with small doses or trials and work up gradually if possible. This is especially the case when detoxifying the body. We provide more free information if you sign up at http://thyroid-adrenal-solutions.com, but we also recommend you work with a holistic practitioner who understands how to safely proceed.

BACKGROUND INFORMATION FOR DIANE CULIK MD

My background a little bit – I went to U of M Medical School and did traditional medicine, I taught residents for about 10 years, and I thought that just by doing screenings I was doing some kind of holistic medicine. Maybe it is a blessing, but I developed, probably about 15 or more years ago, terrible neck pain and headaches.

Every day I would wake up and be in pain and I took aspirin, Motrin and all those things. It would upset my stomach. I didn't want to be a narcotic addict to cover my pain, but I was just in misery and was afraid I was going to end up as a lot of patients are told - to just live with it. This was going to be it.

I had a crazy nurse come in the office and tell me that magnets, if I put them on my neck, would help my pain. I thought that was the stupidest thing in the world - if magnets could help my neck, I would've learned about it at U of M Medical School, because I was a doctor, and she was just a nurse. And boy was I wrong, because the next day my neck and headache were gone!

I woke up and I said to myself "If magnets, which have been researched in Russia and Eastern Europe, and around the world, and there is so much evidence these are safe and natural and effective, and I didn't learn this in medical school, then maybe there's a few other things that they didn't teach us in medical school that could help us," and pretty much everything I do today is what I did not learn in medical school. Let me state that I do use a bit of what I learned there, but most of it is not related to what I am doing these days. So that's where I am coming from today.

THE VIEW FROM 30,000 FEET

So let's start with an overall view as if you were flying high above the scene. This way, you get a picture you can refer to when the detail gets a little more intense later. But our goal for you is to finish this book with the big picture firmly in mind, and to provide you with an actionable list of things you can do to treat your thyroid and adrenals; the actionable list will be given again at the end. There will be tips you can immediately apply to help you feel better and know you are doing the right things for thyroid and adrenal health.

WHAT ARE THE 10 THINGS YOU MUST KNOW ABOUT THYROID DISEASE?

1. Laboratory Tests are often NOT complete
2. Laboratory Tests are often NOT interpreted correctly
3. Laboratory Tests indicate Blood and not Cellular Levels of Thyroid Hormone
4. Physical exam findings may be Significant as an indication of Thyroid Disease
5. Symptoms alone may be Significant as an indication of Thyroid Disease
6. Toxic exposures are significant in evaluating for Thyroid Disease
7. Supplements may be important in supporting normal Thyroid Function
8. Adrenal evaluation and support is important in Thyroid Therapy
9. Food Allergy evaluation is essential in Auto-Immune / Hashimoto's Thyroid Disease
10. Thyroid Prescriptions and Why Natural is best

Number one - thyroid tests are often not complete, the tests that are done, the doctor may come back and say "Hey, I tested you for thyroid, here's the results, they are normal, and you are okay." This may not be true.

Number two - laboratory tests are often not interpreted correctly. So even if they do more than one simple screening test and most do just one test, which is the simple TSH screening test, they then will say, "Yes, I did three or four or even five tests, and you are okay." But this may not be true either, as sometimes they just don't know how to interpret them.

Number three - laboratory tests really indicate what's in your blood, obviously it is a blood test, but this does not really indicate the cellular level of thyroid hormones.

Number four - your physical exam findings may be very significant as an indication of thyroid problems. It is not just the lab tests that count.

Number five - symptoms may also be a very significant indicator of whether you have thyroid disease – so you have to look at other things like how you are feeling as well.

Number six - toxic exposures, and I will be going into detail, are significant in evaluating if you have thyroid disease, what may have caused it, and how.

Number seven - supplements are very important in supporting your normal thyroid and adrenal function, so a lot of things can help you beyond just thyroid hormones.

Number eight - adrenal evaluation is very important in evaluating your thyroid. Your different organs like thyroid and adrenals, they interact and this needs to be addressed.

Number nine - food allergy evaluation is essential in evaluating any Autoimmune or Hashimoto's Thyroid Disease. You've got to do this evaluation.

Number ten – this is about getting on to full thyroid treatment if you need it, and we discuss thyroid prescriptions and why, absolutely, natural thyroid hormone is best for you.

So let's get started. I believe you will find some fascinating tips and secrets along the way.

CHAPTER 1- LABORATORY TESTS ORDERED ARE OFTEN NOT COMPLETE

TSH IS THE GENERAL THYROID TEST USED MOST TODAY

1. Most Doctors only use a TSH test for screening for Thyroid Disease and for monitoring Thyroid dose

2. TSH has a wide range of "normal" and is being re-evaluated and lowered to indicate the healthiest range

3. By itself, TSH testing misses many other test results and evaluations that may indicate Thyroid problems.

Okay, first of all, laboratory tests that are ordered are often not complete - let's start by giving you more detail. Most doctors use only a TSH test, which is a screening test that is commonly recommended. TSH also is used for monitoring the thyroid dose – are you getting enough or too much? But the TSH test has a very wide range of what is normal and is constantly being reevaluated as far as *"what does it mean, this TSH level?"* It is somewhat useful, but used by itself, TSH testing misses other test results that may indicate thyroid problems.

So what are some of the other thyroid tests that can be done?

THYROID BLOOD TESTS EXPLAINED

1. The two Thyroid Hormones are T3 and T4
2. The Free Levels of both are the "Active" levels in blood
3. The Best Measurement is FreeT3, Free T4 and TSH
4. Reverse T3 measures the amount of "inactive" T3 that has been produced to SLOW metabolism
5. Reverse T3 is an isomer or mirror image of regular T3
6. Both are produced from or by T4
7. Reverse T3 production is often triggered by severe diets, stress, starvation, pregnancy, etc.
8. Another cause of high Reverse T3 is Low Iron/or Ferritin

There are two specific thyroid tests that can be used to measure actual thyroid hormone in the blood. Those are T3 and T4, and the "free" level means it is active, not bound thyroid in your blood; this "free" component is the one that's really doing the work. So the best measurements are the free T3, free T4, and then the TSH. The reverse T3 is also something that is very critical and it may be the only thing abnormal and it indicates inactive T3 hormone; it can actually tell you to slow your metabolism, which most people do not want.

Reverse T3 is an isomer or mirror image of what the regular active T3 is; both the regular and reverse T3 are produced from T4, but in reverse T3, your enzyme is shunted and if there is been any severe diet, stress, starvation, pregnancy, it means you develop more reverse T3 and it slows your metabolism.

Several other causes of reverse T3 can be low iron, low ferritin, and cortisol which is either high or low. If you are under a lot of stress, and stress you have had over a long time that has caused adrenal burnout – then that can trigger reverse T3; also insulin and diabetes can cause it, and low B12 may be a trigger. We think that basically this enzyme conversion, which is more common in certain populations and genetics, seems to be a method to preserve the species so we don't die out.

THYROID HORMONES AND REVERSE T3 (RT3) TRIGGERS

1. High Cortisol or Low Cortisol can be a trigger for RT3
2. Insulin Dependent Diabetes can be associated with Elevated RT3
3. Low B12 levels can be another cause of high RT3
4. Reverse T3 seems to be triggered to preserve the species during famine or an individual during starvation
5. With scarce food, an individual lives longer with slowed metabolism and a lower temperature
6. Once an elevated Reverse T3 is triggered in a patient's metabolic pathway, they often maintain slowed metabolism and low temperatures even when food is later abundant and weight is excessive

If you think back 5,000 or 10,000 or even 50,000 years in our history, the main goal is that the body did not starve, so the ability to make T3 probably developed as a species. When food is very scarce and people are going through starvation the people who live the longest are the ones who have triggered this reverse T3, slowed their metabolisms, and lived longer at a lower temperature. So that was great for our ancestors, not starving during a potato famine, but nowadays, once this reverse T3 is triggered it usually stays there – this metabolic pathway continues and has us live in a slowed, cold slow state even when there is lots of food around, or you weigh 300 pounds, no matter what, it often doesn't go back and you stay this way even when there's plenty of food.

THYROID BLOOD TESTING FOR COMPLETENESS

1. Elevated Thyroid Antibodies indicate Auto-Immune Thyroid Disease even with normal T3, T4, and TSH
2. Dr. Hakaru Hashimoto was a Japanese Physician
3. He published a report on this condition in Germany in 1912
*4. He described patients with "**struma lymphomatosa**" which is an intense infiltration of lymphocytes and fibrosis within the thyroid gland seen on biopsy*

Interestingly, when I was talking to Beaumont labs, they said they do not even do reverse T3. I don't know how they get away with it. So the other tests I think are essential are for thyroid antibodies and those can indicate autoimmune disease, even if all the other tests are normal. There is an interesting history here. There was a Dr. Hakaru Hashimoto, a Japanese physician, working in Germany in 1912, over 100 years ago. He published a paper and he described patients he was seeing and he called their condition *"struma lymphomatosa."* He looked at patient's thyroids under the microscope and it showed an intense infiltration of lymphocytes, which are white

28

cells and fibrosis, which is scar tissue in the thyroid gland. This is what he found when he did biopsies.

Thyroid Lab Tests for Hashimoto's Disease

1. "Struma lymphomatosa" was the first recognized auto-immune disease and was later named "Hashimoto's Disease"
2. It is also called "Chronic Lymphocytic Thyroiditis"
3. The blood laboratory tests that must be ordered to evaluate for this condition are:
- Thyroid Peroxidase Antibodies—TPO
- Anti-Thyroglobulin Antibodies—ATG
4. The ATG antibodies can also be elevated with Grave's Disease, Pregnancy, Thyroid Cancer, and Infertility and in people with other auto-immune diseases like Lupus.

This *"struma lymphomatosa"* was the first recognized and described autoimmune disease; now it is called Hashimoto's Disease after Dr. Hashimoto, or other people call it *"chronic lymphocytic thyroiditis,"* which shows inflammation of white cells in the thyroid. A couple tests are important to evaluate for it. The blood laboratory tests that must be ordered to evaluate for this condition are Thyroid Peroxidase Antibodies or TPO and Anti-Thyroglobulin Antibodies, or ATG. Antibodies may also be elevated in Graves' disease (which is the Hyperthyroid condition), and sometimes in pregnancy, thyroid cancer, infertility, and in people with other autoimmune diseases, as in conditions like Lupus.

CHAPTER 2- LABORATORY TESTS ARE OFTEN MISINTERPRETED

TSH LABORATORY TESTS

1. TSH is the screening test most often done by Doctors
2. TSH indicates the "Thyroid Stimulating Hormone" that is released by the Pituitary Gland
3. TSH in circulation stimulates the Thyroid Gland to produce and release more Thyroid Hormone
4. TSH itself is NOT the active thyroid hormone
5. TSH is the brain's thermostatic control for the thyroid
6. When the pituitary senses low thyroid hormone in the blood stream it releases TSH to turn on or turn up Thyroid Hormone Production

So now we have covered all the tests, but how do we know laboratory tests have been interpreted correctly? They are often not. A lot of doctors will just tell you the test was okay, but how do we know whether or not they know what they're talking about? So the TSH is the screening test usually done by doctors. TSH stands for *"thyroid stimulating hormone."* So it's really a hormone not from the thyroid, but one that is released by the pituitary gland. And the thyroid stimulating hormone in circulation stimulates your thyroid gland to produce and release more thyroid hormone. So it is not the active thyroid hormone itself; we really think of it as the brain's thermostatic control to turn off or on the thyroid gland. The pituitary gland senses that you're not getting enough thyroid hormone floating around in the blood and it will trigger the release of TSH and that will turn up the thermostat of the thyroid which in turn will cause more thyroid hormone production.

When TSH is elevated that serves as an indication for a lot of doctors that your brain is trying to get your thyroid to make more hormones, and that may be the first sign of a thyroid problem. So the normal TSH level ranges from .5 to 5.5, and they use that range because they measured 10,000 patients walking around and looking okay, so they thought "these must be normal levels." The problem is it does not reflect the range of those people feeling really great and energetic, and not exhausted and tired. So it is a broad range and one can feel lousy even with so called acceptable numbers.

TSH LEVELS ARE OFTEN NOT INTERPRETED CORRECTLY

1. "Normal" TSH levels range from .5 to 5.5
2. This reflects the wide range of levels in the population
3. It does NOT reflect the range for people who feel great
4. The range includes people with mild thyroid symptoms
5. In 2003 the American Association of Clinical Endocrinologists revised the guidelines
6. Doctors could "consider" treatment for thyroid at lower levels of TSH
7. They recommended that levels above 3.0 **could** indicate thyroid disease with hypothyroid symptoms

But a lot of people don't feel so great in that range, and they do have thyroid symptoms. Not long ago, in 2003, the American Association of Clinical Endocrinologists revised their guidelines and said doctors could now consider and treat thyroid at lower levels of TSH, and that it didn't have to be up at 5.5. They said it could be as low as three and maybe some of those patients could be hypothyroid. Because I'm sure a lot of patients were reading literature online and saying "here are all my symptoms; I must have hypothyroidism," and their numbers weren't that high, and they were demanding that something be done about it. So the Association of Endocrinologists adjusted and said "Well, maybe some of these people may be hypothyroid." But in reality most people I see coming back from the endocrinologists, they say that the endocrinologists stick to that guideline of about .5 to 5.5 as being OK.

TSH LEVELS AND HOLISTIC MEDICINE

1. Many Holistic or Integrative Physicians recognize that TSH levels above 2.0 are often associated with typical symptoms for thyroid disease...AND...
2. These patients often respond very well to treatment with natural thyroid hormones
3. They often will report decreased thyroid symptoms, increased energy, easier weight loss, less dryness and swelling, improved bowel function, etc.
4. TSH levels...IN CONJUNCTION WITH...symptom evaluation is a much more accurate way to determine a diagnosis and treatment plan for Thyroid Disease

So holistic physicians think that probably 2.0 is a pretty good cutoff and above that you have to have a pretty high suspicion that someone may be hypothyroid. What's fascinating is not only that they may be, but when you treat those people with thyroid hormone and other supplements, they often get better. So they seem to have the symptoms, and their levels are above 2.0 and you treat them. They get better and the symptoms go away. To me, it seems like this make sense. Really what you need to expect is that the physician will look at what your levels are in conjunction with what your symptoms are and that is really much more accurate.

DR. BROWNSTEIN'S THYROID BOOK
David Brownstein MD is one of the Top Thyroid Doctors

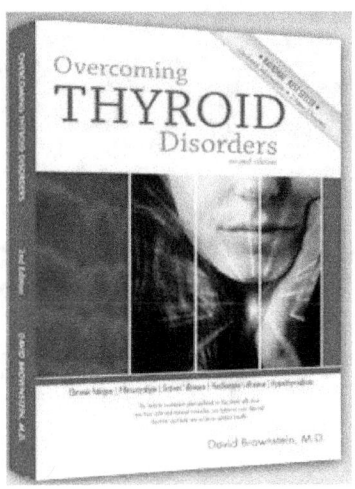

Thyroid Adrenal Secrets Revealed

Hopefully many of you have heard of Dr. Brownstein. He is a local Michigan thyroid doctor, a thyroid expert and a national expert; he has several books, and if you haven't seen his book "Overcoming Thyroid Disorders," it is loaded with information. He has done lots of studies thyroid and iodine, and is a great source of information.

CHAPTER 3- CELLULAR LEVELS OF THYROID HORMONE MAY BE LOW THOUGH BLOOD LEVEL IS HIGH

LAB TESTS INDICATE BLOOD LEVELS AND NOT CELLULAR LEVELS OF THYROID HORMONE

1. Blood test results indicate the levels of Thyroid Hormone in the blood, but not in the tissues and cells
2. Total Thyroid Hormone is mostly bound to proteins such as "Thyroid Binding Globulin"
3. The amount of TBG is often related to hormone levels
4. Birth Control Pills and other hormones increase TBG...and thus more thyroid hormone is tied up and bound to this protein
5. Therefore the "Free" T3 and T4 are more accurate levels than if your doctor orders just T3 and T4

Number three, laboratory tests indicate blood levels, and not cellular levels of thyroid hormone. So thyroid hormone may be strong in the blood, but part of us may be affected because our hormones trigger increased thyroid binding globulin, and this protein binds to thyroid hormones, and prevents them from being active. So if you are on birth control pills or other hormones, this may make your total thyroid levels hard to interpret because more of your thyroid hormone is tightly bound to this protein. Again, that's why we use antibodies, free T3, and free T4 tests as it is another way we can be more accurate in our assessment.

THYROID HORMONE IN THE CELLS

1. When T4 enters a cell an enzyme cleaves off iodine to make the active hormone-T3 (T4-5 Deiodinase)
2. The enzyme that does this relies on adequate zinc and selenium to be effective
3. The enzyme is blocked or poisoned by Mercury
4. Mercury toxicity is often associated with low thyroid
5. Mercury exposure is often from Silver Dental Amalgams
6. People with many silver fillings often have low Thyroid, Fibromyalgia, Chronic Fatigue Syndrome, Parkinson's disease, Alzheimer's disease, etc.

Actually we have T4, which is either what you make in your thyroid gland, or we take Synthroid or Levo-Thyroxine – which is just T4 with four iodines as part of it. In the cells, your body, with an enzyme, cleaves off one of the iodines and converts it to T3 and that is really more important for your metabolism. And the enzyme is called T4 –5 Deiodinase because it takes off iodine. The enzyme that does this relies on zinc and selenium and other factors to be activated and you know it's going to work, but clinically if you have Mercury in your system, Mercury and heavy metals all bind to places they shouldn't and affect things - especially things like iodine - they interfere with its function.

One of the most common places you will find mercury is the silver fillings or amalgams in your mouth. Many people with silver fillings will not only have low thyroid, but if you look at them, they will have fibromyalgia, chronic fatigue, Parkinson's,

Alzheimer's, autoimmune disease, and lots of other problems too.

MERCURY AND DISEASE

1. Mercury is in Flu shots given to adults, children, infants and even pregnant women
2. Mercury is high in fish such as Tuna, Shark, and Halibut
3. The safest fish and only one I eat is Wild Pacific Salmon
4. Mercury has high air concentration around coal processing plants*
*Autism rates are higher in areas with high coal exhaust
* Reference Raymond F Palmer Journal Health and Place, 2008

The other sources of Mercury can be in flu shots and in other vaccinations, not only for us adults, but children, and pregnant women as well. Flu shots have thimerosol, which has mercury, and this is not the safest kind of thing to be exposed to. Mercury is very high in big fish, such as tuna, shark, and halibut. I used to eat a lot of fish, but the only fish I eat anymore is something like wild Pacific Salmon. So farm raised, Atlantic, or other fish - I would not eat it.

Mercury is also present in the air as we are breathing it; it is coming from coal processing plants and factories. One interesting study, done in 2008, mapped out in Texas where the coal burning plants were, and where the highest rates of autism were, and they exactly match, which is quite interesting.

CHAPTER 4- PHYSICAL EXAMS REVEAL MUCH ABOUT THE THYROID

THE PHYSICAL EXAM IS SIGNIFICANT IN DIAGNOSING THYROID DISEASE

1. Certainly Lab tests may help you diagnose Thyroid Disease
2. But the Physical Exam may also be helpful in making a diagnosis
3. Clusters of physical findings make borderline labs or symptoms more likely to indicate Thyroid Problems
4. Dry skin is a common finding in Low Thyroid
5. Patients may constantly be applying oils and yet the skin may feel thickened and even dry and scaly
6. Lateral eyebrow thinning is a common finding
7. Women who don't pluck their eyebrows may find them sparse or need to fill them in with an eyebrow pencil

The physical exam can be quite significant in diagnosing thyroid disease. So we've got the labs, we've looked at the symptoms, but you have got to put in the patient exam too, and a lot of times there may be clusters of physical findings that indicate thyroid problems. I find my patients have dry skin, they may be putting on oil all the time, they may have lateral eye brow thinning, and women who do not pluck their eyebrows find they have to fill their eyebrows in.

PHYSICAL FINDINGS OF THE THYROID GLAND

1. Goiter is an enlargement of the Thyroid Gland - It may be mild or huge
2. Over 100 years ago, the Great Lakes area was called the "Goiter Belt" because so many women had huge goiters
3. The Thyroid Gland enlarges as it tries to absorb more Iodine from the blood stream. (As do the breasts and ovaries with fibrocystic breasts and ovarian cysts)
4. Adding Iodine to salt helped many people in the past
5. The Thyroid Gland usually slowly shrinks when given adequate Iodine supplementation
6. Most endocrinologists just watch goiters enlarge until the Thyroid Hormone Levels are "abnormal"

Goiter, which is enlargement of the thyroid gland, is common and it may be a little or a lot or huge and this part of the country over 100 years ago around the Great Lakes was called the *"Goiter Belt"* because so many women had huge goiters. The thyroid gland tries to get more iodine, because we need iodine to make thyroid hormone, and so it tries to compensate, and like a factory on three shifts it gets bigger and bigger and bigger as it tries to find iodine in the blood stream it can absorb.

So adding iodine to salt in the past helped many people. If you are living in Michigan or the Great Lakes area, and eat only homegrown food you probably lack iodine. Because our state is in the middle of the nation and we don't have any ocean salt, or seaweed, or iodine in our soil, we are very deficient, but if you can supplement iodine or get it from other places, that can help. Unfortunately, and I don't know why this is, many endocrinologists when they see an enlarged thyroid will give the person an ultrasound, will check for nodules, do a biopsy, make sure they don't have cancer, see that the blood test is fine, and say "Okay, we'll see you back here in a year," and the thyroid just keeps getting bigger and bigger and bigger. All you have to do is give the person iodine, and the thyroid gland will shrink down. I don't understand; you don't have to put up with a goiter – it is very easy to treat.

GOITERS-MODERATE AND LARGE
Here are a couple examples of goiters.

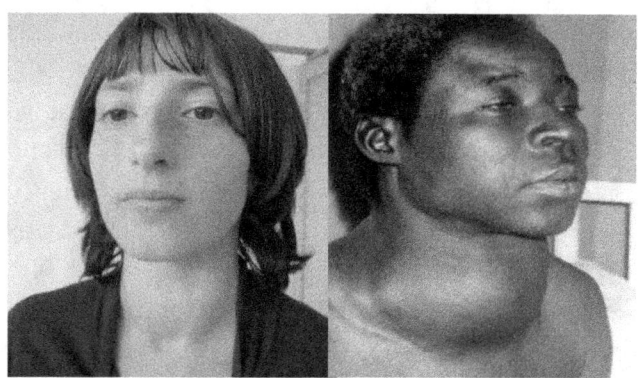

Actually the women on the left, as you can see, hers is pretty prominent so it is not mild, but moderate, and obviously the woman on the right has a much enlarged goiter, and I have seen people walking into my office in these modern times who have goiters that large; it always amazes me.

PHYSICAL FINDINGS IN THYROID DISEASE

1. Hair loss or shedding can be triggered by Low or High Thyroid levels. Hair may be dry and brittle and easily break. Hair may also be lost from the roots
2. The tongue may be swollen with low thyroid conditions
3. The face and especially eye lids may be puffy
4. Hands may be puffy and rings will be tighter
5. Carpel Tunnel symptoms are common with low thyroid and often improve with thyroid supplementation
6. Fingernails may be thin or splitting and easily break

So to speak about other physical findings and thyroid disease - you can have hair loss or shedding which may be triggered by either low or high thyroid levels, hair can be dry, brittle and easily break at the roots, tongue may be puffy with low thyroid, especially when it's severe, face also, and fingers may be puffy and rings will be tight. A purple tone is very common for people with low thyroid.

Carpel tunnel is very common in patients with low thyroid, so sometimes adding a little iodine or extra thyroid and especially B6 can be helpful for carpel tunnel. In addition, fingernails can be brittle and split and break easily.

PHYSICAL FINDINGS IN THYROID DISEASE, CONTINUED

7. The lower legs may often swell with low thyroid
8. Pitting edema may occur with indentation of the skin when pressure is applied with the thumb

9. Severe edema can occur with myxedema
10. Reflexes are often slowed or delayed in the lower legs
11. The Heart rate may be slower than usual in Hypothyroid and sometimes palpitations that will resolve once thyroid hormone is given
12. Certainly fast heart rates and palpitations are common with Hyperthyroid

Other symptoms can be mild to severe edema, sometimes you can stick your thumb into the front part of the legs, and it will just dent in, this is edema. If you measure reflexes, they may be slow or delayed, the heart rate - it may be slow, and I used to think that fast heart rates and palpitations were only in hyperthyroid, which they mainly are, but I've also seen people with low thyroid who get strange palpitations, and if you add adequate iodine or thyroid, the palpitations decrease.

PHYSICAL FINDINGS IN THYROID DISEASE, CONTINUED AGAIN

13. A significant physical finding that you can verify yourself and is an acceptable support for Hypothyroidism by Integrative and Holistic Practitioners is the low morning body or basal temperature.
14. Broda Otto Barnes was born in Missouri in 1906 in a log cabin and he became a Physician who promoted the "Basal Body Temperature Test" to measure first morning temperature as a way to document low thyroid function that he felt was under diagnosed. The body's thermostat is controlled by adequate thyroid.

*15. He had great results with natural desiccated thyroid and adrenal therapies and is accepted only **outside** of traditional Endocrinology circles.*

So one finding you can check all by yourself is to measure your body temperature, and this is something that most integrative, holistic doctors will accept as another clue to thyroid disease or problems. It all started back with Dr. Broda Barnes and he was born in 1906 in a log cabin in Missouri. He became a physician and he promoted that people do a basal body temperature test to measure what their temperature is. He theorized that in all the people and their complaints that there was a lot of under diagnosed low thyroid, and that the low temperature in the morning was an indication that the thyroid was not functioning adequately. So he used natural desiccated thyroid and sometimes hormones and he saw amazing results with his patients - in both their energy and their weight and more. But he unfortunately is not accepted by traditional endocrinologists. Most holistic doctors think he was way ahead of his time.

CHAPTER 5- WHAT ARE SOME SYMPTOMS OF THYROID PROBLEMS?

WEIGHT PROBLEMS AND COLD HANDS

1. Difficulties with weight are very common in Low Thyroid
2. Patients gain weight with no change in Diet and Exercise
3. Or they often "barely" lose weight doing the same diet and exercise that others can successfully lose weight on
4. The metabolism is often different than what it has been...or different compared to others
5. Patients are often "cold" compared to others around them
6. They have ice cold hands, wear socks to bed, wear sweaters and jackets, and turn up the heat, even when others are warm in the same environment

Please understand that symptoms alone can be significant as an indication of thyroid disease. Other thyroid symptoms that some people might have include weight problems. It's very common with low thyroid, though not always as I have seen some people who are very thin, but often people will find they are gaining weight without touching anything. They say, "I am eating the same, and exercising the same, but not losing weight like others."

They are out there dieting, they are hardly eating anything, they are doing exercise and everybody else is losing weight like crazy, but nothing is working for them. So there is some discrepancy in everything they are doing. Patients are also cold, their hands may be cold, their feet may be cold, they may wear socks to bed, certainly in the winter, sometimes even in the summer, and they are putting on jackets and coats when no one else is doing so.

MOOD ISSUES AND FATIGUE

7. Mood issues are common symptoms in Hypothyroidism
8. Patients have fatigue and symptoms of depression or irritability or often with memory and focus
9. They often struggle to get through the day and do daily activities that had once been easy
10. Fatigue is common no matter how much sleep they get
11. Low thyroid patients can sleep 10 hours and still be tired
12. They may often take naps after work or during the day on weekends, and later fall asleep watching TV

Mood issues can be common in low thyroid patients because sometimes they're so tired and exhausted that they feel depressed and irritable; they have trouble with memory and focus. They may just struggle to get through the day; it's so much harder to do this when they have fatigue, they may feel that no matter how much sleep they get they are still tired, even after 10 hours sleep.

It's hard to get up, it's hard to function, they may need to come home from work and take naps in the evening and they may fall asleep in front of the TV, etc. Now these are not the only problems, obviously, but these are ones that are quite common with low thyroid conditions.

Sluggish Bowels and Infertility

13. Bowel problems are often a chronic symptom with low thyroid
14. For some patients this is a new problem but others complain they have been "sluggish" their whole lives
15. Some say their bowels are "normal" but they take frequent or daily laxatives to keep them that way
16. Patients with auto-immune thyroid disease may have loose stools, diarrhea, gas, bloat or been told they have "IBS"
17. Periods are often irregular, light, or heavy, skipped, or stop or have Amenorrhea and no periods
18. Infertility may often be caused by subtle low thyroid

Bowel problems - I hear this all the time from people with low thyroid, and some patients say it's relatively new, while others say "I have been that way all my life, so it doesn't mean anything." They may complain "I am sluggish" or they may say "I am fine," but they're taking thyroid hormone or laxatives or prunes, on and on and on, just trying to keep themselves going. And they think this is normal because that's the way they've been for a long time.

If they have autoimmune thyroid problems often they will have associated food allergies and they may have constipation or diarrhea. They may have been told they have IBS, or they may have gas or bloating, so it's not just constipation, especially in the autoimmune patients. Periods are often irregular, they may be light or heavy or close or far apart; they may have cramping or they may have amenorrhea. So they can be all over the map. Oftentimes, they're just not having the regular typical period.

In addition, infertility is certainly very common, especially with low thyroid. If it's borderline thyroid, it may be picked up, but I've seen a lot of women that are just slightly off and you get them on some thyroid and possibly iodine, and they get pregnant very quickly. So you have to warn them, if they are not pregnant and they thought they couldn't become so that they just might get pregnant and very easily.

Chapter 6- Toxic Exposures are Significant in Evaluating Thyroid Disease

Mercury and Dentistry

1. Mercury is a Toxic Heavy Metal associated with Thyroid Disease
2. One of the most common exposures is Silver Fillings
3. One of the first things to evaluate in someone with Fatigue, Depression, or Cold Intolerance is if they now or previously had mercury fillings or if mercury is hidden under a dental crown
4. The most common symptom related to Mercury is Depression
5. Dentists have the highest rates of Depression and Suicide of any Profession. Dentists and Dental assistants are exposed to inhaling mercury vapor when cleaning and drilling teeth

Number six, toxic exposures – there are a lot of problems related to toxins with low thyroid. Most relevant I think is mercury, and I mention silver fillings and one of the first things I look at in a patient is are they fatigued, depressed, do they have cold intolerance, have they now or in the past had silver fillings, or do they have mercury under a dental crown? One of the most common symptoms from mercury toxicity is depression, and if you think about it, dentists have the highest rate of depression and suicide of any profession. Dental assistants and dentists are exposed to mercury as they are taking out fillings and putting in fillings, cleaning, drilling teeth, even if they are holistic dentists who don't put in silver fillings anymore, they are probably taking care of people who have these fillings and are drilling and taking them out.

MERCURY'S EFFECT AND OTHER SOURCES OF MERCURY

6. Mercury blocks deiodination of T4 to T3
7. This affects low cellular T3 and fatigue, depression, high cholesterol, heart disease and erratic heat regulation result
8. Mercury interferes with the production of ATP producing enzymes and again causes fatigue and slow metabolism
9. Mercury can also be found in waterproof mascara, fungicides, some hair dyes, preservatives in vaccines- Thimerosol, hemorrhoidal medicines, yellow, vermillion and cinnabar paint pigments, mildew resistant pains, gardening chemicals, and...fluorescent light bulbs

Dentists also get exposed to mercury over many years and it can cause problems, certainly also for the dental hygienists as they have a lot of pregnancy and fertility problems too. So mercury not only blocks the enzyme that converts T4 to T3 and causes low cellular T3 and fatigue and depression, but also because of the low thyroid, patients develop high cholesterol and heart disease, and there may be heat deregulation. Mercury even affects our bodies' mitochondria, and ATP, which is the energy production in the cells so people may have fatigue and slow metabolism.

49

So a lot of people have correlated that chronic fatigue and fibromyalgia and thyroid patients may have a lot in common, because they all have mercury toxicity and there may be a lot of overlap in their list of symptoms. Mercury not only does the things we describe, but is found in mascara, fungicides, hair dyes, preservatives and vaccines, with thimerosol being the big ingredient in most vaccinations. It is also found in hemorrhoid medications, paint pigments, mildew resistant paints, gardening chemicals and even fluorescent light bulbs. You will find that if these light bulbs break, you can get mercury exposure.

PFOA – ANOTHER THYROID TOXIN

1. PFOA has been shown to be toxic to the Thyroid Gland
2. Perfluoro-Octanoic Acid is in non-stick pans
3. People with the highest levels of PFOA in their blood have:
- Double the incidence of Thyroid Disease
- Increased Infertility and Chronic Kidney Disease
4. PFOA is a Toxicant and a Carcinogen and is in 98 % of people's blood in US
5. PFOA is not only common in Teflon Pans
6. It is also commonly used to line Microwave Popcorn bags and the popcorn is coated with it that you then eat*
(*Ref. Wikipedia)

Another interesting toxin is PFOA and this has been shown in a lot of studies to be toxic to the thyroid, and is something to try and avoid. It is called Perflouro-Octanoic Acid, and it is in non-stick pans, and people with the highest levels of this acid in their blood have double the incidence of thyroid disease, have increased risk for infertility and kidney disease, and increased risk of other problems as well.

It's known that this is a toxin, a carcinogen, and when they have done studies, they found 98% of us have some in our blood, so it is everywhere, but we want to have it affect us as little as possible. So not only get rid of your Teflon pans, but interestingly enough, it is commonly used to line microwave popcorn bags, so the popcorn is loaded with PFOA, which can affect your thyroid. Is also found in stain resistant carpets and carpet cleaning liquids – which is a problem if you get your carpet cleaned regularly, and I just read today on Mary Shoman's website that there is a lawsuit being leveled against DuPont, who makes PFOA, and there's been a big increase in disease in some areas because they're discharging PFOA into the water.

SOY IS ANOTHER TOXIN IN THYROID DISEASE

1. Soy is toxic to the Thyroid Gland
2. Many people consume soy milk, cheese, burgers, and tofu but don't realize it is hidden in protein shakes, dressings, and many processed foods
3. The "Whole Soy Story" by Kaayla Daniel, PhD, blows the lid off the dogma that Soy is a health food.
4. Soy is related to: Malnutrition, Digestive Distress, Cognitive Decline, Reproductive Disorders, Infertility, Birth Defects, Immune System Disease, and Heart Disease, Cancer and Thyroid Dysfunction

Another interesting toxin is soy – which is very toxic to the thyroid gland and other things. Many people knowingly consume soy when they buy and eat soy milk, cheese, burgers, or tofu, but it's hidden in so many other foods including protein shakes. A lot of people I know drink protein shakes, they don't know if the protein is soy or whey or rice protein, and soy is also in salad dressings. Most salad dressings at the store have plenty of it. It's also in many processed foods that use soy as an ingredient.

A fabulous book written by Kayla Daniel, PhD, is called "The Whole Soy Story," and blows the lid off the idea that soy is a health food. She has shown, with lots of research, that soy is related to malnutrition, digestive distress, cognitive decline, reproductive disorders, infertility, birth defects, heart disease, cancer, and thyroid dysfunction.

COULD SOY BE USED AS AN AID TO CELIBACY?

According to Kaayla Daniel, it may be and she writes…
"Can soy be used as an aid to celibacy?" Is it true that Zen monks eat soy because naughty behavior goes down when tofu consumption goes up? Do Japanese wives feed unfaithful husbands extra helpings of soy? Could politicians with the "zipper problem" keep their naughty bits better under control if they consumed enough soy? Anecdotally the answer is yes and a fair amount of science backs it up"
From the Journal "Nutrition" comes a case study of a 19 year old heterosexual man who began consuming lots of soy after becoming vegan and soon experienced a loss of libido and erectile dysfunction.

So this was really cute from her book – "Can soy be used as an aid to celibacy?" (Hillary says so....) And one little story from the Journal "Nutrition" talks about a 19-year-old heterosexual man who consumed a lot of soy after he became vegan and soon experienced a loss of libido and erectile dysfunction – at 19. So if you are not getting rid of soy for your thyroid health, you might want to consider getting rid of it for the health of all your other body parts.

Soy Toxicity

1. Soybeans contain plant estrogens – isoflavones
2. The isoflavones resemble estradiol and bind to estrogen receptors and then interfere with the body's production of its own estrogen, testosterone, etc.
3. Isoflavones genistein and daidzein are potent inhibitors of thyroid peroxidase (TPO) the enzyme involved with the synthesis of T3 and T4
4. They block the iodinization of the amino acid tyrosine which is critical in thyroid hormone production

Soy toxicity – soybeans contain plant estrogens called isoflavones, and these resemble estradiol and bind to estrogen receptors. So it interferes with your own estrogen by binding to these estrogen receptors. Isoflavones are called genistein and daidzein and they are potent inhibitors of thyroid peroxidase or TPO, and this is the enzyme that helps make thyroid hormone, the T3 and T4. So when you are eating soy you are blocking thyroid production. They block the iodinization of the amino acid tyrosine, which is critical to make thyroid hormone.

CAUSES OF THYROID CANCER

1. Soy has been implicated in the increased incidence of Thyroid Cancer

2. Other toxic exposures that have been shown to increase Thyroid Cancer include:

* Exposure to Radiation...especially when young. (Children in the 1940's and 50's had radiation to their necks and "enlarged thymus" for prevention of crib death. This resulted in destruction of their thyroids and later development of thyroid cancer.)

* Mercury, Fluoride, Plastics, Pesticides, Dioxins, Solvents, Low Iodine Intake, Estrogen mimickers in commercial meats and produce also implicated in Thyroid Cancer cases

Soy and thyroid cancer - you see an increased risk of thyroid cancer for lots of reasons, but one reason they have shown in the literature is for the use of soy. Another reason, if you have not heard of it, is back in the 1940s and 50s doctors used to radiate children's necks, they would use X-Rays and they'd see an enlarged thymus gland. They did this for prevention of crib death in new babies. So they shrunk the thymus down, and this resulted in thymus destruction and years later, you're seeing development of thyroid problems, thyroid disease, hypothyroidism and thyroid cancer from all that radiation when these people were infants.

Other causes of cancer can be mercury, fluoride, plastics, pesticides, dioxins, solvents, low iodine intake and estrogen mimickers in commercial meats and produce. There's a great story about Dr.

Brownstein, where he had a woman with thyroid cancer who traditional doctors could not help, and he gave her massive doses of iodine and seemed to resolve her thyroid cancer.

FLUORIDE TOXICITY

1. Fluoride is Toxic to the Thyroid Gland
2. It interferes with the body utilizing Iodine since it is a competing Halide
3. It is in our water, toothpaste and mouthwash
4. Holistic Dentists have shown that ingested Fluoride is toxic to early tooth development and causes pigmentation and damage called "dental fluorosis"
5. Fluoride is toxic to the kidneys, brain, and causes bone cancer risk
6. 97% of Western Europe has chosen Fluoride Free Water
7. Fluoride is a toxic byproduct added to water
8. It should be avoided, filtered, removed, and eliminated from our Tap Water and Toothpastes

Fluoride toxicity – fluoride is toxic to the thyroid gland. It interferes with the body utilizing iodine, which it needs because it is a halide. The problem is our government places fluoride in the water and it's also in our mouthwashes and toothpaste and people say is good for us, but it's not. Holistic dentists have shown that ingested fluoride is toxic to early tooth development, causes dark pigmentation and can cause irregularities, permutation and a condition called dental fluorosis.

Fluoride is also toxic to the kidneys and brain and can even cause bone cancer risk. If you talk to the

Europeans, who studied it, and are doing things not because their local governments are making money buying or selling fluoride for the water, 97% of Western Europe has decided and has chosen to have fluoride free water – I wonder why? Fluoride is a toxic byproduct added to our water and we all pay for it, but it really should be filtered, avoided, removed and eliminated from tap water and dental treatments, and also eliminated from toothpaste and mouthwash.

#6-Dental Fluorosis

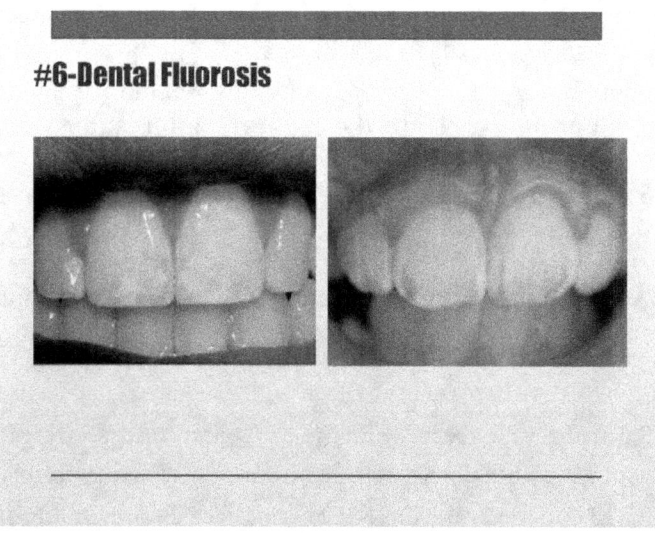

Here are a couple pictures where you can see a little irregularity in color and a little bit of brownish stain on the teeth, and below is another picture which shows even more severe damage where the teeth may be mottled and even brown from the fluoride.

#6-Dental Fluorosis

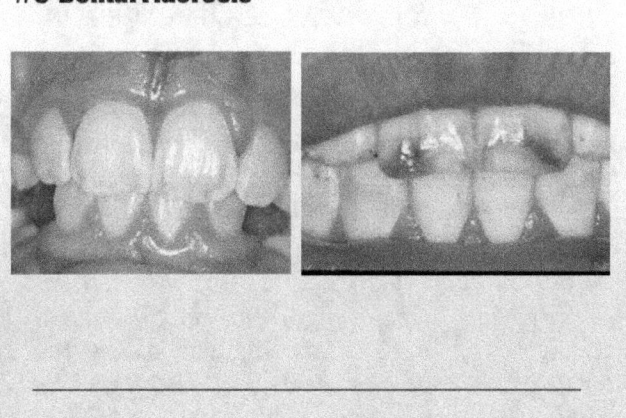

FLUORIDE TOXICITY TO THE THYROID

"Fluoride Changes The Shape Of The Enzymes So That They No Longer Fit. Since enzymes are proteins, once they've been changed, they're now foreign-looking. The body now treats them as invaders, even though they're part of that body. This is known as an autoimmune situation – the body attacks itself. Another way to look at it: enzymes are long-chain proteins held in certain shapes. Hydrogen bonds are the Velcro strips that hold the enzyme in a certain shape. Fluoride comes along and hydrolyzes the enzyme – it cuts the Velcro strips away. The shape collapses. No more is it an enzyme; now it's just a foreign protein."

So fluoride is toxic and changes the shape of the enzymes, and destroys the bonds in the enzymes, changes the shapes so they don't work, and they look like foreign protein.

57

FLUORIDE TOXICITY WAS DOCUMENTED IN THE 1920S

"The Effects of Fluoride on the Thyroid Gland" – By Dr Barry Durrant-Peatfield, Medical Advisor to Thyroid UK 9-9-4. It has been known since the latter of the 19th century that certain communities, notably in Argentina, India and Turkey were chronically ill, with premature aging, arthritis, mental retardation, and infertility; and high levels of natural fluorides in the water were responsible. Not only was it clear that the fluoride was having a general effect on the health of the community, but in the early 1920s, Goldemberg, working in Argentina showed that fluoride was displacing iodine; thus compounding the damage and rendering the community also hypothyroid from iodine deficiency.

Here are some interesting facts about the effects of fluoride in the 19th century, in Argentina and Turkey; they knew that many of these areas had certain communities that were chronically ill with premature aging, arthritis, mental retardation, infertility. Why? This was because they had extra fluoride in the water naturally. It was clear that fluoride was very detrimental to the community and not only did it cause these diseases, but they knew then that it displaced iodine and caused people to be hypothyroid. So this was back in the 1920s.

FLUORIDE TOXICITY SHOWN AGAIN IN 1930S

*FLOURIDE IS HIGHLY DAMAGING TO THE THYROID GLAND—"This was the basis of the research in the 1930s of: May, Litzka, Gorlitzer von Mundy, who used fluoride preparations to treat over-active thyroid illness. Their patients either drank fluoridated water, swallowed fluoride pills or were bathed in fluoridated bath water. **<u>Their thyroid function was as a result, greatly depressed.</u>** The use in 1937 of fluorotyrosine for this purpose showed how effective this treatment was; but the effectiveness was difficult to predict and many patients suffered total thyroid loss. **So it was given a new role and received a new name, Pardinon. It was marketed not for over-active thyroid disease, but as a pesticide.** (Note the manufacturer of fluorotyrosine was IG Farben who also made sarin, a gas used in World War II)."*

*It is a little known fact that **fluoride compounds were added to the drinking water of prisoners to keep them docile and inhibit questioning of authority, both in Nazi prison camps in World War II and in the Soviet gulags in Siberia. "This** bit of history illustrates the fact that fluorides are dangerous in general and in particular highly damaging to the thyroid gland. While it is unlikely that it will be disputed that fluorides are toxic—let us be reminded that they are Schedule 2 Poisons under the Poisons Act of 1972, the matter in dispute is the level of toxicity attributable to given amounts; in today's context the degree of damage caused by given concentrations in the water supply."*

So the research showed that they were using fluoride to actually treat people who were hyperthyroid, they would give them fluoridated water, fluoridated pills to depress the hyperactive thyroid. The problem is they could not control it, and some people completely lost thyroid function, so they decided to eliminate it as a treatment for thyroid. The manufacturer of this thyroid toxin, who also made sarin gas, then used this compound as a pesticide to kill bugs.

One of the especially interesting things I read about fluoride is that it was used in the Nazi prison camps and the Soviet Gulags in Siberia, and put in the prisoner's drinking water to keep them docile, so they would not question authority. It made them very tired and weak. So history illustrates that fluoride is dangerous in general and in particular very bad for the thyroid gland, but that alone doesn't show just how much is going to make you docile, and how much is going to destroy your thyroid and how much will just make you tired, and low temperature. But all in all, it is best to avoid it. It also should be noted that fluorides are schedule two poisons under the Poison Act of 1972.

OTHER HALOGEN TOXICITIES TO THE THYROID

1. Besides Fluoride, the other Halogens that compete for binding sites with Iodine include chlorine and bromine
2. Chlorine is used to kill bacteria in tap water...and ultimately also kills the good bacteria in the gut
3. Bromine is in Bromo-Seltzer, brominated flour and thus most baked goods, Hot Tubs, Mountain Dew
4. Halogens compete for the binding with the few molecules of Iodine we may have ingested
5. Dr. Brownstein has demonstrated in thousands of patients in Michigan that 96% are deficient in Iodine

6. When given large doses of Iodine, they excrete the toxic Halides such as Fluoride and Bromine

So what other halogens are bad besides fluoride? It has been found that chlorine and bromine are also toxins. Chlorine is in our water, and if you drink it, it kills off the good bacteria in your gut, as well as the bad bacteria. So you have to repopulate the good bacteria with probiotics. Bromine, found in Bromo-Seltzer, is also in flour, all the flour you have bought the last few years has bromine in it to make it fluffy, so if you're eating regular bread, baked goods, or pastries, you are getting bromine, and it is going to be interfering with iodine and therefore toxic to your thyroid.

Bromine is also found in Mountain Dew. So these halogens compete for iodine and what Dr. Brownstein mentions is that he found that 96% of people in Michigan are low on iodine and he gave them large doses of iodine and he checked their urine. A lot of these halides, like bromine, fluoride, come out, so you can detoxify yourself from these toxins.

Toxins, Yeast and Low Thyroid

1. There is a high association between Yeast and Hypothyroid patients
2. Yeast may be releasing chemical toxins that interfere with Thyroid hormone effectiveness
3. People with low thyroid production seem more susceptible to recurrent yeast infections
4. "The Yeast Connection and the Woman" by Dr. Crook reports that many common symptoms of fatigue,

allergies, IBS, diarrhea, bloat, asthma, cough, sneeze, itch, headaches, sinus congestion, muscle aches, and sore throat may all be related to low grade yeast.
5. Treating yeast through herbs, supplements, nutrition and sometimes prescription methods helps in "Thyroid" and other patients.

Yeast, commonly called Candida, is a toxin associated with low thyroid. Yeast cells growing in you release a chemical toxin that interferes with your thyroid hormone's effectiveness.   People who have low thyroid are often more susceptible to yeast, and they often have mercury in their bodies. A great book "The Yeast Connection and the Woman" by Dr. Crook says that many of the symptoms of yeast are often similar to thyroid problems - fatigue, allergies, IBS, cough, sneeze, itch, muscle aches, sore throat.

A lot of these can be caused by yeast. And if you treat the yeast infection, certainly through a low glycemic diet, or take herbs, supplements, or talk to a nutritionist, (and sometimes prescriptions will help), you can help energy and often support active thyroid function.

DIABESITY AND HYPOTHYROIDISM OFTEN HAVE A COMMON TRIGGER

(From Toxins in foods and the environment per Dr. Mark Hyman, a Family Physician and Holistic expert)
"Scientists have shown that toxins cause increases in glucose, cholesterol, and fatty liver, and slow down your thyroid function.   They may also cause an increase in appetite and signals that control hunger.

Toxins make you fat and must be addressed in any treatment program for diabesity."
For info and supplements see: http://abcwellness.healthylivingshop.com

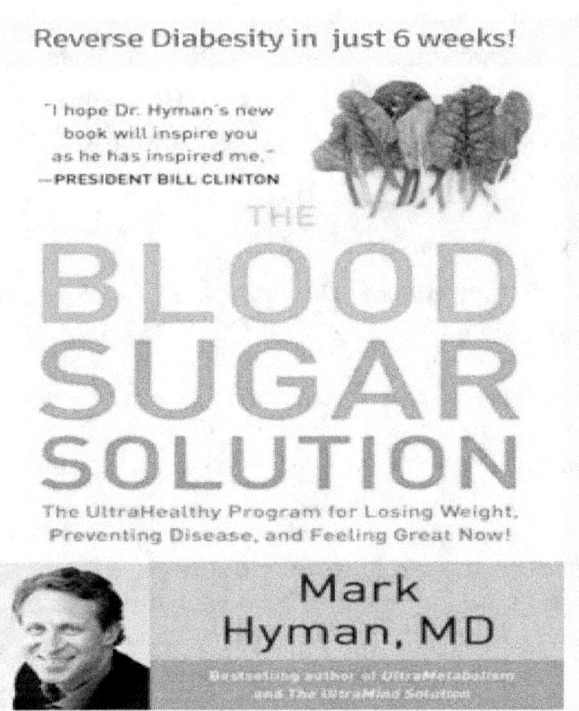

A condition that is similar and related to this is diabesity. Dr. Mark Hyman is one of the top doctors in the country and he wrote this book called "The Blood Sugar Solution" which talks about "Diabesity" a term he coined for diabetes and obesity, and he shows it is related to hypothyroidism because of toxins in the environment. I love how he says he knows he is a holistic doctor because all the patients coming to his office bring a "whole list of problems."

So anyway, he says scientists have shown that toxins cause an increase in glucose, cholesterol and fatty liver and slow down your thyroid function. They may also cause an increase in appetite and signals which control hunger. Toxins make you fat and must be addressed in any program for diabesity, which is similar for the treatment of thyroid.

TOXINS AND DISEASE

Toxins that affect Diseases like Hypothyroidism, Obesity, Diabetes, Hypertension, Elevated Cholesterol and Cancer include: Mercury and Heavy Metals, Aluminum in deodorants and pans, Teflon, Yeast, Bacterial overgrowth in the gut, Fluoride, Bromine and Chlorine, Pesticides in most foods, Plastics from water bottles and dishes and wraps, Hydrogenated oils in almost everything from chips to fries, to crackers, to baked goods and pastries, to fried meats, to salad dressings, to almost everything you eat in a restaurant that is fried or stir fried or cooked. Avoid soybean, corn, safflower, canola, oils, etc. Use only coconut oil to cook and olive oil for cold foods.

We've covered a lot of toxins and their effect on the thyroid – and we looked at diseases like hypothyroidism, obesity, diabesity, hypertension, elevated cholesterol, and cancer. We also looked at mercury and heavy metals, but it's also aluminum in deodorants - there is aluminum in some vaccines which is toxic, and Teflon pans, yeast, bacterial overgrowth - because you're killing of the good bacteria in the gut, fluoride, bromine, and chlorine.

You want to minimize pesticides in most foods, and eat organic when possible. Avoid plastic water bottles; you should purchase a filter for your water. Hydrogenated oils are in almost everything you eat from chips to fries to crackers to baked goods and pastries. This is so it will stay fresh on the shelf for years.

Also a problem is fried meats, salad dressings, and almost everything you eat in a restaurant that is fried or stir-fried or cooked. Avoid soybean, corn, safflower and all the other bad oils. Use only coconut oil to cook and olive oil for cold foods. A lot of times you go to the grocery store and you look at the ingredients in a food and you see that olive oil is practically the last ingredient on the list.

TOXINS AND INFLAMMATION

1. Thyroid and Weight Gain - If you have any desire to lose weight you must avoid inflammatory foods
2. Sugar and Hydrogenated oils and Artificial Sweeteners are always necessary to avoid.
3. Artificial sweeteners cause 200% increased obesity and 57% increased Diabetes.
4. Wheat flour and Dairy products cause inflammation in most people.
5. To test if you are actually allergic requires IgG or IgA blood testing and only IgE is positive if you have hives or acute allergic reaction like a peanut allergy.

Thyroid Adrenal Secrets Revealed

Toxins and inflammation affect thyroid and weight gain. If you have any concern or interest in losing weight the things you must avoid are sugar, hydrogenated oil, and artificial sweeteners. A study just came out that said artificial sweeteners like NutraSweet, and others, caused 200% increased obesity and 57% increased diabetes. You don't want this.

The other things that many, many of us are allergic to are wheat flour and dairy products and I am just amazed by how many people show inflammation from these things. You can test for them to see if you're allergic with IgG or IGA blood tests, but not your allergist's skin tests; these IGE test won't help you unless you have a peanut allergy or an asthma condition.

CHAPTER 7- SUPPLEMENTS TO SUPPORT THYROID AND ADRENALS

NUTRIENTS, ADAPTOGENIC HERBS, THYROID HORMONES, IODINE

1. Many Nutrients are essential for adequate thyroid hormone production
These include: Iodine, Zinc, Selenium, Tyrosine as well as Vitamins A, B, C, E and CoQ10
2. Adrenal support is also essential – Adaptogenic Herbs can be used
3. Adaptogenic Herbs are very helpful for Hypo or Hyper-Thyroid Conditions
4. Thyroid Hormones are composed of 3 or 4 Iodine molecules in T3 and T4 and Iodine has been known to be essential for normal thyroid activity for well over 100 years

So many nutrients are important for your thyroid. These include iodine, zinc, selenium, and tyrosine as well as vitamins A, B, C, E and CoQ10, which is helpful. Adrenal support is essential; adaptogenic herbs are very good for both hypo and hyper or low and high thyroid conditions. So we know we need three or four iodine molecules in our T3 and T4 and iodine has been known to be essential to normal thyroid activity for over 100 years. It just somehow got lost by the doctors practicing today.

IODINE DEFICIENCY NEEDS TO BE ADDRESSED WORLD-WIDE

1. Worldwide Iodine Deficiency affects about 2 Billion People
2. It is the leading cause of preventable mental retardation
3. Cretinism is stunted growth and brain development from Iodine Deficiency
4. It is a congenital deficiency of Thyroid Hormone usually due to the mother's Hypothyroidism and low Iodine
5. Goiter and Cretinism was common around the Great Lakes and Pacific Northwest in the early 20th century
6. David Murray Cowie was a professor of Pediatrics at the University of Michigan - He encouraged the Swiss practice of adding Iodine to table and cooking salt

It is interesting that world-wide iodine deficiency affects about 2 billion people and it is the main cause of preventable mental retardation in the world. The leading cause is simply lack of iodine which is simple, and cheap to solve.

Cretinism is a stunted growth of the body and brain from iodine deficiency and usually it is caused from being born in a mother who is low on iodine and thyroid hormones. And goiter and cretinism were common in this part of the country around the Great Lakes back 100 years ago, and in the Pacific Northwest.

David Murray was a professor of pediatrics at the University Michigan, and he decided from all these kids he was seeing that we should maybe take up the practice of what they were doing in Switzerland at the time which was adding iodine to salt. If you were not getting it in the food grown locally, you needed to have some way, as a country, to get more iodine. So, on May 1, 1924, iodized salt was first sold in Michigan, and by the fall of that year, iodine was being put into the salt across the entire country.

USING IODINE TO SUPPORT THE THYROID

On May 1, 1924 Iodized salt was sold commercially in Michigan. By the fall of 1924, Morton Salt Company began distributing iodized salt nationally.
See the worldwide initiative: Preventing Brain Damage from Iodine Deficiency
www.iodinenetwork.net

There is a great website called www.iodinenetwork.net that is a worldwide fund that talks about iodine deficiency. Many countries still have problems with goiter and cretinism. Holistic practitioners recommend replicating the iodine intake of the Japanese.

The Japanese have the longest life span for men and women of any country in the world, and for the developed nations, they have the lowest rate of breast cancer. They, on average, take in at least 12,500 micrograms a day of iodine because they eat seaweed. They put seaweed on their soil as a fertilizer, and they also get a huge amount of iodine in their diets. And most Japanese look good, feel good, are healthy, and live a long time.

Our government recommends only 150 µg of iodine, which is in a teaspoon of salt, that is, if you eat a teaspoon of regular salt a day. Some people don't even get this small amount, as they don't even eat regular salt. The problem is the Government put this amount of iodine in the salt before they put fluoride in our water, before we had bromine in our breads and flours, before we had all these other toxic chemicals we are now exposed to.

(It is recommended you not eat white salt as it has been stripped of its nutrients. Use a quality Celtic or Himalayan Sea Salt, pink or gray, and get your iodine separately from seaweed, kelp or other sources.)

IODINE IS OFTEN FORGOTTEN, IGNORED AND FEARED

Holistic Practitioners recommend replicating the Iodine intake of the Japanese who have the longest life expectancy and lowest Breast Cancer rates in the world
-This means at least 12,500mcg/day rather than our government's recommended 150 mcg in 1 tsp. salt
Iodine is often forgotten and ignored and feared in this country. It is essential for our bodies.
Dr. Brownstein explains in detail.
-Over 95% tested-inadequate Iodine
-2005 US study showed 16.8 % with severe Iodine Deficiency
-Increased risk for Infertility and Miscarriage and Birth Defects if a woman is even able to get pregnant

-10% of Women develop goiter after pregnancy as Iodine depleted
-13.5 % Lower IQ scores in children with low iodine levels
-29% of World Population lives in areas deficient in Iodine in the soil

So iodine is very important, and is often forgotten and ignored. When it was tested for by Dr. Brownstein, he says his patients tested very low. A 2005 study showed 16.8% of the U.S. had a severe iodine deficiency.

There is increased risk of infertility, miscarriage, birth defects, if you can even get pregnant. 10 percent of women develop goiter after pregnancy, because the baby sucked all the iodine out of the mother. And 13.5% lower IQs scores resulted in children with low iodine levels. Lastly, 29% of the world population has low iodine in their soil.

Iodine is the "Universal Medicine" for prevention of Cancer, Diabetes, Heart Disease and Radiation Protection, per Dr. Mark Sircus, with forward by Dr. Brownstein.

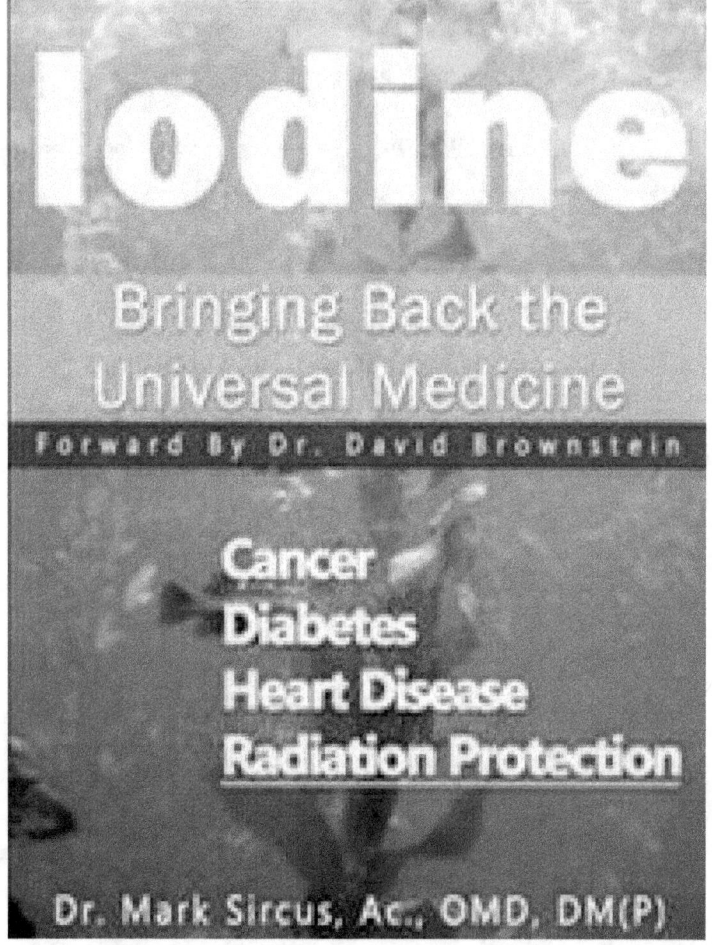

Another great book, by Dr Mark Sircus, with a forward by Dr. Brownstein, is called "Iodine: Bringing Back the Universal Medicine." It says in this book that iodine is not only for cancer, diabetes, heart disease, but also radiation protection, especially after incidents like the Japanese fallout.

CHAPTER 8- ADRENAL EVALUATION AND SUPPORT IMPORTANT TO THYROID THERAPY

ADRENALS AFFECT THE THYROID AND SHOULD BE TESTED

1. The Adrenals work in concert with the Thyroid Gland
2. If either one is not functioning well it will thus effect the functioning of the other one
3. Blood levels of Cortisol, DHEA-S, and Pregnenolone can be measured
4. A set of 4 Saliva tests for adrenal over 24 hours is the most accurate way to evaluate adrenal function

Adrenal evaluation and support is important to thyroid therapy. The adrenals work in concert with the thyroid gland. They sit on top of the kidneys and react with the thyroid, and if either one is not working, you will not have maximal function of each. You can do a blood level test for cortisol, DHEA–S, and Pregnenolone, and for more accuracy you can test saliva over 24 hours for a patient to see how it is cycling during the day.

SYMPTOMS OF ADRENAL INSUFFICIENCY

In 1998, Dr. James Wilson coined the term "Adrenal Fatigue" – see www.adrenalfatigue.org , characterized by:

73

1. Fatigue and Exhaustion for no reason
2. Trouble getting up in the Morning
3. Need Coffee, Coke, Salt or Sugar to try and energize
4. Difficulty with Sleep
5. Decreased Mood and Depression
6. Low Libido
7. Run Down and Difficulty with Handling Stress
8. Decreased Immunity

A great person, Dr. James Wilson coined the term *adrenal fatigue* in 1998, which still has been not accepted by endocrinologists, but he saw a very significant set of consistent symptoms in his patients which he could treat with multiple modalities. He has a website at www.adrenalfatigue.org.

What he saw is that many different people had symptoms like fatigue, exhaustion, trouble getting up in the morning, need for a coke or coffee, salt, or sugar to get moving, they had difficulty with sleep, their mood was low, they were depressed, their libido was bottomed out, they were run down, they were having trouble handling stress, and had decreased immunity – a whole list of troubling symptoms.

ADRENAL MANAGEMENT TOOLS

1. Nutrition
2. Supplements, Vitamin C, Natural Sea Salt
3. Adaptogenic Herbs
4. Adequate Deep Sleep
5. Activity and Exercise
6. Adrenal Hormones
7. Stress Management
8. Energy Therapies: EFT and Emotion Code

He found that with consistent management through many modalities this condition could be improved. Definitely nutrition is critical, (that is eliminating the bad, and putting in the good), having adequate supplements like natural sea salt with minerals, vitamin C, melatonin, adaptogenic herbs, adequate deep sleep, activity and exercise, and oftentimes adrenal hormones, doing stress management, and even energy therapies, like yoga, EFT and emotion code.

One of my associates does emotion code and releases trapped emotions, she does this in our office and has had great success with that.

Chapter 9- Food Allergies, Hashimoto's Disease Facts and Therapy

FOOD ALLERGY EVALUATIONS

1. Essential in Auto-Immune Thyroid or Hashimoto's Disease

2. Hashimoto's Disease is usually triggered by an inflammatory insult to the Thyroid Gland that triggers the Auto-Immune Reaction. This could be viral, infection, heavy metal or other toxins.

3. Everyone I have evaluated with Hashimoto's Disease has allergic antibodies to foods, usually wheat and dairy.

4. Everyone I have tested with Lupus, Rheumatoid Arthritis and Vitiligo and other auto-immune conditions has one or often several food allergies.

5. Diagnosis of the allergy is essential for control and therapy and minimizes risk of other diseases.

Food allergy evaluation is essential if you have autoimmune disease, whether it be thyroid or any place else. Now Hashimoto's is triggered by an insult to the thyroid gland; this could be viral, infection, heavy metals or other toxins. And although sometimes it is triggered by a virus or infection, I have found that everyone tested that has high thyroid antibodies has food allergies, and often many other things.

Everyone I tested for Lupus, Rheumatoid arthritis, and Vitiligo and other autoimmune conditions has one or many food allergies. We are becoming more and more allergic to the food we eat. I don't know why, but I see it, and when people recognize it and go off those foods, I have seen Lupus go away, I've seen Rheumatoid Arthritis go away, and this is without drugs, without taking toxic drugs that are going to destroy your immune system, people can get better. So it's hard to find out what the cause is and people have to be willing to remove those things from their diet that are causing problems.

PHYSICAL FINDINGS IN HASHIMOTO'S DISEASE

1. The Thyroid exam may show an enlarged, firm and lobulated gland
2. Also the Thyroid exam may be perfectly Normal
3. Thyroid Peroxidase Antibodies (TPO) and/or Thyroglobulin Antibodies may be elevated
4. Hashimoto's Disease often results in inflammation and destruction of the gland and inadequate thyroid hormone production and <u>Hypo</u>thyroid symptoms
5. Episodic <u>Hyper</u>thyroid symptoms may occur with antibody destruction of the cells, stimulating excessive release of thyroid hormone

So in Hashimoto's disease you may have an enlarged, firm, and lobulated thyroid gland, or it may feel normal, but the thyroid peroxidase antibodies, TPO's are elevated, or thyroglobulin antibodies are elevated.

So you may have inflammation, and destruction of the thyroid; eventually all patients have low thyroid, or hypothyroidism, but during that time when there is inflammation and antibodies, there is destruction of the thyroid cells and that releases thyroid hormone which is accompanied by hyperthyroid symptoms.

SYMPTOMS OF AUTO-IMMUNE HASHIMOTO'S DISEASE

1. Symptoms may be very similar to non-autoimmune thyroid disease:
Weight Gain, Hot and/or Cold, Fatigue, Anxiety, Panic attacks, Depression, Slow or Fast Heart Rate
2. Hashimoto's is 5-10 times more common in women
3. Only 1 of 8 with Food allergies may have GI symptoms such as IBS, heartburn, abdominal bloat, gas, indigestion, constipation or diarrhea
4. Symptoms may only be acne, headaches, migraines, brain fog, joint pains, muscle aches, neuropathy, rash, wheeze etc as a clue to food allergies and subsequent auto-immune Thyroid Disease

So basically these people have a lot of the same symptoms that a regular hypothyroid person has, they may be cold and tired, have weight gain, fatigue, anxiety, panic, depressions, but with Hashimoto's - it is interesting. Hashimoto's is five times more common in women and even though I say most of them have food allergies, they may have G.I. symptoms such as abdominal pain, irritable bowel syndrome, heartburn, gas, indigestion, constipation or diarrhea.

Commonly I see acne, headaches, migraines, and brain fog, muscle aches, joint pains, neuropathy, ADD, rashes, all kinds of other symptoms throughout the whole body. And this may serve as a signal that there is some kind of inflammation going on.

More Information on Hashimoto's Disease

1. The Genetic predisposition for Hashimoto's is evident in Twin Studies
2. Identical or Monozygotic Twins have 80% concordance
3. 38-55% of Identical Twins have similar symptoms
4. Therefore, some may have the antibodies and not symptoms
5. Non-Identical Twins have much less occurrence together
6. Hashimoto's is common in families with other auto-immune diseases such as: Celiac, Vitiligo, Pernicious Anemia, Rheumatoid Arthritis, Lupus, and Diabetes

So you need to do food allergy testing to find and eliminate triggers. Sometimes you do a panel with 96 different food allergies with a few drops of blood, and I've seen some people that are allergic to like 23 things – that's not all that common. But that inflammation triggers bowel inflammation and leaky gut, yeast, and lower energies and it's a vicious cycle as more things become inflamed, and you become reactive to more things.

Hashimoto's is more evident in twins. In 80% of identical twins, if one has Hashimoto's, the other will, and even though they don't all have symptoms, they will both have high rates of antibodies, and certainly they will have some genetic predisposition.

If you have in the family one person with an autoimmune disease like Hashimoto's, another may have diabetes and another may have lupus, another may have rheumatoid, or they may have Vitiligo, so there's a whole spectrum of diseases that somehow genetically some of us are more predisposed to.

AUTO-IMMUNE THYROID THERAPY

1. Food Allergy Testing and Eliminate Triggers
2. Essential to test gluten and dairy and egg
3. May require a 96 panel or more blood test for other foods
4. Avoid inflammatory foods in general-sugars, Tran's fats
5. Gut inflammation from allergies leads to "Leaky Gut"
6. Soothe and heal the Intestinal tract with probiotics, prebiotics, Glutamine, Amino Acids, Phyto-nutrients
7. Use anti-inflammatory Omega 3s as Fish or Krill Oils
8. Use Coconut oils in cooking/heat and baking, sautéing

So you have to assume a leaky gut besides the reactive foods, you must give the patient adequate nutrients and Omega threes, make them use good oils, glutamine, amino acids, probiotics, lots of things that calm down the inflammation and amazingly, the thyroid antibodies, oftentimes they will fall or decrease because you've got to the source or cause of that inflammation.

Chapter 10- Thyroid Treatment and Why Natural Thyroid Hormone is Best

NATURAL THYROID HORMONE FACTS

1. Natural thyroid is usually derived from actual thyroid glands, and has been used for therapy over 100 years
2. It is standardized and blood levels are consistent
3. It contains T4, T3, and even T2 and T1
4. Your body relies on a perfect environment of nutrients and avoidance of toxins for conversion of T4 to T3
5. Simple T4 therapy like Synthroid or Levothyroxine usually is NOT adequate to treat low thyroid SYMPTOMS, even if your blood tests or TSH is OK
6. Our bodies require active T3 in the cells for energy

Let's talk about thyroid treatment and why I believe natural thyroid hormone is best. Absolutely, I think that natural thyroid hormone is best; if you talk to a lot of doctors they say it is not consistent, but it has been used for over 100 years. It is very standardized, they have to have it be very consistent, most of these contain not only T4 like Synthroid, but also T3 and a little bit of the others like T2.

Our bodies rely on all these nutrients because of all the toxicities and heavy metals and deficiencies, most of us don't have enough cellular conversion of T4 to T3. So you need to take one with T3. (This is assuming you have properly detoxified your body, and have added all the supplements like iodine, vitamins and minerals and everything else, and you are still showing low thyroid symptoms. Always keep trying to heal yourself to the point where you can go without taking anything if possible.)

NATURAL THYROID TREATMENT DIRECTIONS

1. Thyroid symptoms and lab tests are stable if thyroid medication is taken consistently
2. Usually this is best done the first thing in the morning on an empty stomach
3. I recommend people keep their thyroid pills in the bathroom and take them with water on awakening, as long as there is no concern about kids or pets getting them
4. If forgotten, take anytime and with any food – it is better to take thyroid medicine than not taking at all

So I really believe for most of us that simple T4 is not going to work, it is not going to be effective enough to get good results for you and you really need to take T3 to get good levels in your cells so that thyroid symptoms and lab tests are stable. But to do this you have to take your medication consistently.

We have found Natural Hormones really do work, people have good results. It is probably best to take them in the morning on an empty stomach, but if you forget, take them anyway. Just put them somewhere safe so your dogs or kids won't get to them.

MARY SHOMAN'S WEBSITE AND BATTLE CRY

1. Mary Shoman is a nationally recognized thyroid expert and author with web site www.thyroid.about.com

2. "60 million Americans have Thyroid Disease and most don't know they do." Of those diagnosed the majority don't even feel well", until they are treated effectively and usually with natural thyroid.

3. "We're patients, not lab values" is her motto and battle cry.

If you haven't seen www.thyroid.about.com, Mary Shoman is not a doctor, she's not a chiropractor, she's just a thyroid patient, but she has tons of information and questionnaires about thyroid and constant updates for her readers about what to do and what to take when it comes to the thyroid.

She says 60 million Americans have thyroid disease, and most don't know it. For those who are diagnosed most of them don't even feel better until they are effectively treated and usually with Natural Thyroid Hormones. She says "You are patients, not lab values!" and that's been her motto and her battle cry.

NATURAL THYROID HORMONE OPTIONS

1. Armour Thyroid, NatureThroid and WestThroid are Natural desiccated thyroid hormones

2. They can be effective, but for many people the T4 may still lag behind on blood tests

3. These thyroid medications have a set ratio of T3 to T4 in their production

4. When the T3 is maximized the T4 may still be too low, or the reverse can happen in some people

So what are some of the options when it comes to Natural Thyroid Hormones? Well, you can get Armour Thyroid, Nature-Throid, and WestThroid as natural desiccated thyroid hormones and for some out there this is quite okay.

But for many people they may lag behind on the blood tests for T4. I try to optimize both the T4 and the T3 when I treat patients. So they have a set ratio on how much to give and interestingly enough a lot of times T3 will be pretty good, but T4 lags behind and is something to consider as people aren't yet feeling great.

So if you get a compounded thyroid hormone, we can precisely dose it so both of those levels are good, and you are not doing too much, and causing palpitations or tremors, but you're getting a full effect of the energy. So you're getting the maximum benefit at very precise dosing with a compound combination.

Compounding Thyroid pills through a Compounding Pharmacy such as "Physician's Compounding Pharmacy" allows an EXACT dosing for both the T3 and T4 - Maximal benefit for Thyroid dosing is easiest this way.

CONCLUSION

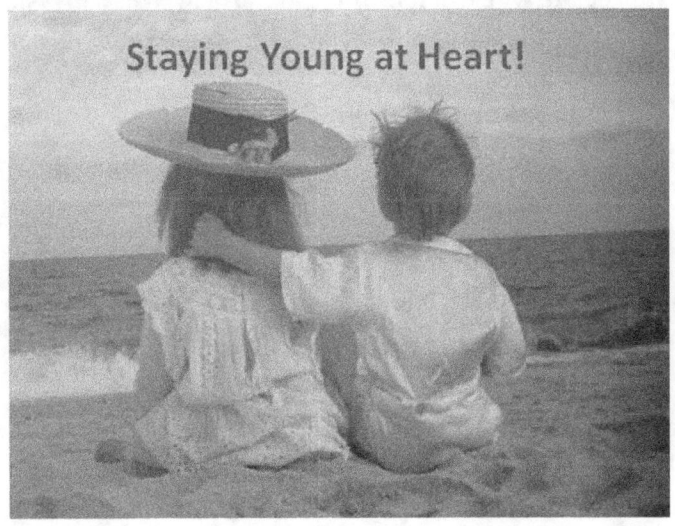

So overall, my summary is to always stay active and young at heart, always trust your body for what it needs to feel healthier and if you don't feel healthy, look for options on how to improve your health, because there are a lot of websites, magazines, books, out there that are fantastic, and there's so much information that you can access and learn about that can help you succeed.

This is not the end of the book by far as for your benefit we have included a number of bonus chapters that may bring more answers you seek. Please excuse us if a few of these chapters contain sales information.

We sell only limited numbers of these products anyways, but we hope they might bring you valuable health tips. Please feel no obligation to buy. We appreciate you reading our material. We will ask, however, that if you liked this book, please consider leaving a positive review on Amazon.

Thank-you for reading, and I hope you find success and happiness on your road to true health!

Diane Culik MD
ABC Wellness

Bonus- An Actionable Plan

NOW YOU KNOW MORE....BUT WHAT TO DO?

You can start with this list below. If you find this helpful, and want further detailed guidance, each step is expanded on in the book below this list:

25 STEPS FOR YOUR THYROID AND ADRENALS

1. Complete Lab Testing for the Thyroid
2. Complete Physical exam for Thyroid
3. Review and complete Thyroid questionnaire of symptoms
4. Measure your morning body temperature (ok over 97.8)
5. Food Allergy testing if any thyroid antibodies or symptoms
6. Nutritionist Consultation if Food Allergies documented
7. Heavy Metal testing if Mercury Amalgams, Fish intake, or other exposures or neurologic symptoms
8. Vitamin testing for Zinc, Selenium, B Vitamins, etc
9. Spectracell Testing for Intracellular Nutrient Levels
10. Avoid Soy, Fluoride, Bromine, Chlorine, PFOAs, Teflon
11. Avoid Mercury Amalgams, Toxic Vaccinations and Fish
12. Adequate Sleep: use Melatonin or Herbal Teas as needed
13. Adequate Vitamin C 2-4,000/day reasonable
14. Use unprocessed sea salt for adrenals
15. Detoxify the Liver with Herbs and Nutrients
16. Heavy Metal Detox if Elevated Levels
17. Herbal and Nutritionist Therapy to Cleanse Yeast/Candida

18. Iodine at 12.5 mg/day or more for Thyroid, Breast, Ovaries
19. Vitamin D to keep 25 Hydroxy-D levels at 50-80
20. Add Vitamins and Minerals that are deficient
21. Adaptogenic Herbs and Natural Hormones when needed
22. Saliva Testing for Adrenals
23. Absolutely avoid food allergens – if allergies, do full food allergy panel
24. Probiotics and Nutrients for gut healing
25. Natural Thyroid Hormone therapy as indicated

Finally, don't forget to Laugh – it's the best medicine of all.

FREE Gift – This entire eBook is attached at the end of this book as a free gift to you!

Or you can go to the website listed below and we will send you this eBook free of charge!

Also, you can see a free video on thyroid adrenal care and for an even more comprehensive video based program, and for free gifts and articles on thyroid and adrenals by email, please visit and sign up at http://thyroid-adrenal-solutions.com

ABC Wellness "Simple Steps to Better Health!"

Did You Like This Book?

Let everyone know by posting a review on Amazon.

<u>Just click here and it will take you directly to the reviews page</u>:

Other Books by ABC Wellness in the "Simple Steps to Better Health" Series:

Thyroid, Adrenals and Weightloss: **The eBook "<u>Thyroid Adrenal Weightloss Solutions</u>" is live in the Kindle Store and is available for purchase.** This book also has the 25 steps.

How to Heal Yourself Naturally: **The eBook "<u>Heal Your Whole Body Naturally</u>" is live at Amazon and is available for purchase.**

Lose Pounds Quickly by Overcoming Obstacles to Weightloss: **The eBook "<u>The ABC Wellness Weightloss Pyramid</u>" is live at Amazon and is available for purchase.**

Acid Reflux or GERD: **The eBook "<u>Acid Reflux Relief Now</u>" is live at Amazon and is available for purchase.**

Anti-Aging Secrets: **The eBook "<u>Insider Bio Identical Hormone Secrets and</u>**

<u>More</u>" is live at Amazon and is available for purchase.

Longevity and Anti-Aging Advice: **The eBook "<u>How to Live to 100 – Top Dos and Don'ts</u>" is live in the Kindle Store and is available for purchase.**

Please forgive us if any sites referenced in our eBooks are not operational when you visit them, and please try back later, as they may be under construction. Thank-you!

BONUS: TOP WEIGHTLOSS TIPS TO CONSIDER

We realize that not all of you will want to lose weight, but we have included these tips for everybody because they deal with healthy eating habits. Hopefully some of the steps you have taken above have removed the thyroid and/or adrenals as obstacles to weight loss, but we wanted to add a few more tips to help you get healthier and lose pounds. You may know some of these already, but it never hurts to go over them again. Let's list out some top tips:

1. Reduce your sugar intake to 25 grams or less per day. Yes, hard to do, but if you can, you will find losing weight a lot easier. Please don't underestimate the power of this step – this one point can let you have success losing weight! Many years ago, people consumed a fraction of the sugar they do today. If you are ever not feeling well, cut your sugar immediately. It can work miracles. Give this a try and keep track of your sugar intake and your body weight for the next 7 days and keep the grams as low as possible. You may be amazed at the result.

2. Get rid of the pop – if you must have it, drink it by itself as a treat away from meals. Not diet pop either, if you are going to give in, drink the regular kind, hopefully with real sugar and not high fructose corn syrup.

3. Avoid corn products of all kinds that have corn that has been genetically modified.

4. Eat only when you are hungry, and just enough to fill you up, skip the desserts.

5. Consider skipping meals occasionally, maybe even look into possibility of short term fasting. It has been proven in studies of mice that calorie restriction increases longevity, and it makes sense that humans can benefit from this strategy too. Think about it – it gives the organs a rest and the whole system a chance to purge toxins. The best and easiest way may be to have supper, begin your fast, and fast until the next day's dinnertime for a quick 24 hour fast. You might even do this once a week. Or try going on a 2 meal a day strategy, eating at around noon and 6 pm, or any time when you feel hungry. This will let your blood sugar stabilize.

6. Try coconut oil – a tablespoon or so a day.

7. Concentrate on eating home grown or organic vegetables, with some lean protein. Look into the Weston Price kind of diet. This is a superb way to stay healthy.

8. Avoid refined, processed foods, eat as close to nature as possible.

9. Take a spoonful of quality flax oil and fish oil every day or two. Experiment by taking cod liver oil for a few weeks and see if you benefit. You may be surprised.

10. Resolve digestive issues with apple cider vinegar – just an ounce in a small glass, 3 or 4 ounces of water. A good choice is Bragg's Apple Cider Vinegar with the "Mother."

11. Here is one of the biggest secrets ever, and perhaps this should have been listed first. Instead of worrying so much about losing weight, concentrate on increasing your strength and therefore your muscle mass as well. You can in a matter of a few months of real lifting transform your body in an amazing way. Of course, this is hard work, and you should clear with a doctor that you are ready for handling a heavy exercise schedule. This is not just for men anymore; many women have experienced the thrill of a new way of life through weightlifting. When you carry increase muscle mass around, your resting metabolic rate is raised, and you burn off excess weight easier. You also worry a lot less about diet, but by paying attention to both, you can change radically and quickly.

After saying all the above, we do have to make a statement to clarify things. We realize heavy lifting is not for everyone, just those who have real motivation for change. So, for most, plan to exercise moderately, even 30 minutes 3 days a week, and that will help boost metabolism; 5 or 6 days is better if you can handle it. Use weight lifting exercises as well as aerobics. Building muscle means you will burn more calories, and feel better too. You increase the oxygen getting into the cells, and you will also be able to fight off infections more rapidly too.

ABC Wellness "Simple Steps to Better Health!"

These are just a few tips to supplement other diet and or weightloss programs you may follow. Actually, the point is that if you go through all or even some of these steps, you may find yourself losing weight if you hit on one or more points or obstacles that need attention.

For those wishing to learn some great secrets and do not like the exercise approach, we do recommend the following program; to see a video, click link: <u>Beyond Diet Program</u>.

Bonus: Resource List

For your convenience, we have listed sources for supplements below. There is absolutely no obligation to buy, but we do appreciate it if you do. No matter where you make your purchase, please remember to buy only high quality items – your body deserves the best.

Here are sites you can go to for thyroid, adrenal, detoxification, hormonal and weight loss helpers that Dr. Culik approves of and are of high quality:

www.drculik.com (and go to the upper bar for NUTRITION)

- ThyroMedica Plus for enhancing thyroid function
  AdrenaMed for maximizing adrenal function
- T-100 includes freeze dried thyroid and adrenal gland plus minerals and herbals
- Weight loss, CLA Trim, MCT Oil to improve metabolic function, and Total Vegan Chocolate and Vanilla

Shakes that are not only gluten but dairy free so no whey or Soy
* Dual-Tox for maximizing liver cleansing for energy and weight loss

www.purecapspro.com/drculik. For vitamins and minerals and natural mood therapies

www.mydoterra.com/abcwellness. For essential oils for mood, hormonal support, for weight loss, detoxing, yeast infections and other infections including Lyme disease

Http://dianeculik.isagenix.com. For complete protein drinks either whey or nondairy, IsaCleanse for detox and weight loss...Ionix supreme for adaptogenic support of thyroid and adrenals...e+. Energy drink for natural boost of energy and metabolism

www.purerxo.com/ABCwellness

www.dssorders.com/ABCWellness
HCPC374WELCOME, DC374, $100

Shop anytime online
Website:
Registration Code:
☑ Order by Phone toll free: **877-846-7122**, 8:00-6:00 CST
☑ Enroll in Auto Ship for automatic deliveries — FREE shipping and 5% off.
☑ Rewards: Purchases earn points for future savings

Thyroid Adrenal Secrets Revealed

- ☑ Free shipping on orders over
- ☑ Coupon: Save 10% on your first order →

Bonus: Check Out These Special Offers!

We have found some other programs you may be interested in. The ones listed next are now available – just click to see the presentations on each topic on the following page. There is no obligation to buy, but these may give you the results you seek:

- <u>The Beyond Diet Program</u>: All Natural Diet, Click to view presentation
- <u>Total Wellness Cleanse</u>: Natural Food Based Cleanse!
- <u>Coconut Oil</u>: Boost your Metabolism and Get a Free Book on use with your Purchase!
- <u>Sleep Program</u>: Learn how to get better sleep!
- <u>Bodylastics</u>: Inexpensive, Excellent Exercise Program with Bands!
- <u>Candida</u>: Stop yeast infections now!
- <u>Hypothyroidism Exercise Revolution</u>: Better way to exercise if you are hypothyroid

To supplement the material above, we have included some questions and answers from a recent session at ABC Wellness. We hope you find the answers informative and helpful. Some of the information you may know already, but look them over and see if you can benefit.

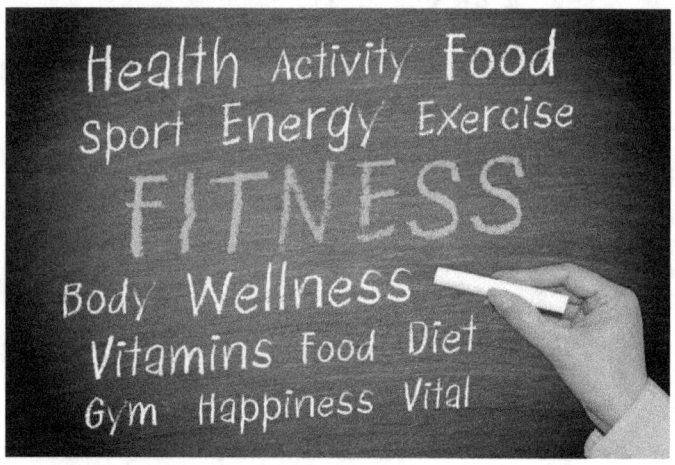

BONUS: QUESTION AND ANSWER SESSION NUMBER ONE

1) The bio identical or natural progesterone cream containers, they have a warning from California that it is cancerous, you say it fights against cancer. Why are they saying it is cancerous?
2) How do you know if there's bromine in your bread, is it listed in the ingredients? Why would they put bromine in the bread?
3) About bromine, how do you know what your level is and if it is a problem, do you measure it in the blood and how do you know if you are toxic?
4) I use a swimming pool for exercise; what about the chemicals, is it safe to do this?
5) My blood pressure runs low. What can you do about that; what can you do to bring it up?
6) What is the ideal testosterone level a person should be at?
7) If you have been diagnosed with a food sensitivity or food allergy, is that diagnosis for life?
8) Are you testing for iodine and how do you test for it?
9) Can you give your opinion on the "eating for your blood type" kind of diet?

The bio identical or natural progesterone cream containers, they have a warning from California that it is cancerous, you say it fights against cancer. Why are they saying it is cancerous?

(This following statement was made by a representative present from a compounding pharmacy.) "A lot of times, people make things that are similar to some other product. They are saying it is similar to something that another company makes, another commercially available product, which in this case is the synthetic hormone product and they are doing this just to cover themselves. In my opinion, it is just basically ignorance, not knowing the difference between the synthetic and the natural or bio identical hormones. The bio identical or natural hormones are protective; the synthetic or "horse" hormones are not."

How do you know if there's bromine in your bread, is it listed in the ingredients? Why would they put bromine in the bread?

From what I've read and what the experts say it can be in any flour, and it is listed on the package. I am not sure why society would do this; it makes the bread light, and fluffy, yes, and this may be the reason they use it, but it is toxic.

About bromine, how do you know what your level is and if it is a problem, do you measure it in the blood and how do you know if you are toxic?

I don't know of any regular lab that tests for bromine levels, but I think Dr. Brownstein measures it in the urine, and sends it out to a lab, a special lab. He has given mega-doses of iodine to people and measures their urine, and has seen a lot of bromine and fluoride coming out, so he knows he is detoxing those things from these people.

I use a swimming pool for exercise; what about the chemicals, is it safe to do this?

Well, a lot of times there is chlorine in the pool, you can smell the chlorine, and that does the same kind of thing as bromine to your body. It is toxic. I would not know what to do about those chemical levels, other than asking the person in charge of your pool to take care that toxic chemicals are not used. (Someone in the audience mentioned that it is possible to get a salt water system for your pool. Maybe that would eliminate the problem.)

My blood pressure runs low. What can you do about that; what can you do to bring it up?

You can try eating more protein, more meat, but some people's blood pressure just normally and naturally runs a bit lower than others. So this is something you want to take up with your doctor. For a lot of people, a little bit lower blood pressure is not a problem.

What is the ideal testosterone level a person should be at?

It varies with the lab, but most labs give a range, sometimes from like 200 to 800, but really, for men you really want to be more like 500 to 800 - that kind of range. For women, it varies with the lab, and a lot of times with supplementation with something like estradiol, that number may be more like 20 or 15 or 10, maybe 15 is a good number. To clarify that, we can say that the testosterone range for women is 2-45 for total and .2 to 3.7 for free and unbound

103

testosterone...usually mid-range is good at 15-30 total and .5 to 3.0 for free testosterone.

If you have been diagnosed with a food sensitivity or food allergy, is that diagnosis for life?

Some of those allergies are probably life-long from what I've seen. If it is gluten, it probably is life-long. Maybe with some other items you may not be sensitive for life if it is not an IGE kind of allergy - that is a peanut kind of allergy. So maybe then it is reversible. But if you are allergic to wheat or dairy, one of those kinds of items, you may have leaky gut and inflammation going on, and you may become allergic to other things. However, if you heal the gut and get rid of the inflammation, you might eventually be able to go back to those food items over time. Maybe six months or a year later you can test to see how you do, see if it is okay to eat those foods again.

What happens if you ignore your food sensitivities?

If you don't address the food sensitivities you have, a lot of people over time will become more and more sensitive to other foods and they will develop more autoimmune disease - heart disease, cancer, things like that. One of the interesting statistics I have heard, from a gluten expert, is that if people even have a touch of gluten even once a month, they have more than six times the increased risk of death from all causes over the years. And this could be from eating just a little bit of gluten even as small as a fingernail sized portion. This is comparing them to someone who is not gluten sensitive. But if they are gluten sensitive and avoid all gluten, then their risk of death is cut in half and this was based on following people for many years.

Are you testing for iodine and how do you test for it?

I used to do what Dr. Brownstein did and I used to give 4 capsules of iodine to people to test the level of iodine in their urine. Eventually I gave up this testing because almost everyone I tested was iodine deficient, that is 95% or more, and Dr. Brownstein found these same kinds of numbers. This is why I recommend people supplement to the Japanese level of iodine found in their diets, which is like 12,500 micro grams or 12.5 mg. So I recommend these higher levels unless a person has thyroid or breast cancer, or thyroid cysts or something of that nature.

Can you give your opinion on the "eating for your blood type" kind of diet?

Well, I have several patients who have used that kind of diet and found some success. Some swear by it, but I've not personally followed these people over time to know whether it is valid or not. Certainly for some people, it seems to work. It is absolutely not a bad thing, though, and may be helpful to people.

BONUS: QUESTION AND ANSWER SESSION NUMBER TWO

1) Will this information be made available to us?

2) Have you written a book?

3) Do your handouts come with the recommended dosages of the supplements?

4) I am curious, artificial sweeteners, and diet pop, I have heard a lot about aspartame, can you comment on this?

5) What about Stevia?

6) I have a question, on one of your slides; you say that vaccinations are causing a problem. What is your take on that?

7) My main question was about vaccinations for babies and children as there has been a lot a controversy lately – what is your take on this?

8) I have a daughter with autism, and they gave her a last vaccine when she was two years old. At first I didn't care much about these stories, and I did not believe it. But she turned two years old and she got the vaccine, and she regressed. My second daughter, I did not do any vaccinations until she was a little older, not when she was a baby, but when she was older, in her preteens and teens, but I was very conflicted about it, any thoughts on this?

9) Why do all these hospitals require vaccinations?

Start Answers:

Will this information be made available to us?

We are working now to prepare it and it probably will be in an e-book form, maybe a video and it may be posted on our websites, you can check it www.drculik.com and http://www.abcwellnessnews.com. But you can also go to Amazon.com and type Dr. Culik and you will find my books that way.

Have you written a book?

We have posted a few e-books on Amazon.com so far, and we have some video presentations made of some of our talks, one on thyroid, one on bio identical hormones, one on acid reflux disease, you can Google, Amazon, and Dr. Culik and find my books that way, or go to Amazon Kindle Books and type Dr. Culik.

Do your handouts come with the recommended dosages of the supplements?

The e-books and the videos will have the dosages as I recommended them, you can check again on Amazon.com.

I am curious, artificial sweeteners, and diet pop, I have heard a lot about aspartame, can you comment on this?

Well, NutraSweet and Aspartame, they change the name so people don't recognize it, and it causes neurological damage, when they first tested it caused holes in the rat's brains, it never should've been on the market –

there was a big controversy. So Searle made it and then hired a couple of the FDA people who were investigating them, hired them over to work at Searle, bought them out, and the FDA dropped the case.

What about Stevia?

Stevia is natural, and xylitol's okay. No NutraSweet or Splenda.

I have a question, on one of your slides; you say that vaccinations are causing a problem. What is your take on that?

When I started out, I thought the best thing I was doing for patients and I wrote an article about it, was getting them to have flu shots. I no longer recommend flu shots, if patients want them, I will send them somewhere. But I haven't gotten flu shots in years. Flu shots still even today have mercury in them, although they have taken steps to pull the thimerosol out, it is still in some of them.

My main question was about vaccinations for babies and children as there has been a lot a controversy lately – what is your take on this?

Many of the children I see, and I don't see that many kids, I mainly see people middle age and older, usually the kids I see, usually their parents don't want vaccinations for them, and they are looking for a doctor who will support them in that. My receptionist has never had a vaccination on her three kids and even before she started with me. I am recommending that she probably start a few now. But I've seen a lot of healthy kids who have not had vaccinations and I definitely don't think you need to get the hepatitis B shot at birth, because it's for people who are going to be sexually active or shooting up drugs. It was going to be for teenagers, and they couldn't get them to do it. So the schedule, the amount of vaccinations, I talked to many, many families at the autism conference I went to and almost to a person they said at age 13 months or 18 months their kid stop talking after their vaccines, this came out in story after story after story. They absolutely believe it, that it is the vaccinations.

I have a daughter with autism, and they gave her a last vaccine when she was two years old. At first I didn't care much about these stories, and I did not believe it. But she turned two years old and she got the vaccine, and she regressed. My second daughter, I did not do any vaccinations until she was a little older, not when she was a baby, but when she was older, in her preteens and teens, but I was very conflicted about it, any thoughts on this?

There's a website called www.cdautism.org, for chlorine dioxide, and there is a woman in Mexico, I think she's American, but she's in Mexico who is curing kids using chlorine dioxide. Using it orally, and as enemas plus nutrients, and absolutely no wheat, no dairy, but using probiotics, and she is normalizing kids, absolutely, back to normal.

Thyroid Adrenal Secrets Revealed

Why do all these hospitals require vaccinations?

I have written a lot of letters trying to get people out of it, but it is such an accepted practice, you do what you can.

BONUS: QUESTION AND ANSWER SESSION NUMBER THREE

1) What is the Paleo diet?
2) There's been a lot of in the research about Carnitine, I hear that it helps for energy and weight loss, but lately it seems the bad news about Carnitine, you heard anything?
3) So you went through a lot of information here – how does one get all this information if we were not able to take all the notes?
4) What do you think about Spirulina? Is a good for you?
5) And look at the fluoride; they put it in toothpaste – what you think of that?
6) How do you get good water?

What is the Paleo diet?

Basically they are looking at what did our ancestors eat, not our grandparents, but what the cavemen ate, what was natural. They are addressing the question of should we all be vegetarians, or should we all eat meat, or both? What kind of vegetables and meat?

Their theory is that our ancestors ate a mix of proteins and vegetables that they would just pull and harvest. So they were not doing grains, they were not farmers out farming wheat and corn or rice or something. So they ate meat, and they obviously ate a lot of vegetables, and they basically had all kinds of combinations of those things.

The more you can do, as most people think, of the wild, the organic, the grass fed kinds of proteins, (although sometimes they're very high in protein), and less of the more complex grains and vegetables the better. So no potatoes, no beans either. Basically, they are doing the asparagus and a slab of meat, that kind of thing.

There's been a lot of in the research about Carnitine, I hear that it helps for energy and weight loss, but lately it seems there has been bad news about Carnitine, have you heard anything?

Yes, as I just said some people are just going to eat their Carnitine and their red meat – I just saw an email on that. But obviously there's a difference of opinion there. Listen to the experts – I don't know the complete answer there – it might be good to do some research on the topic.

So you went through a lot of information here – how does one get all this information if we were not able to take all the notes?

Well, I have a handout that you get after you fill out your evaluation form. This handout has a summary of the resources, the websites, the books, the magazines, the types of test, the things to look for, and if you put your email on there when the information is pulled together, I think we're going to be sending out an email summary, so you can just go on that document online and click links, so that will make it easier and we will probably posting it on my website at www.drculik.com or at www.abcwellnessnews.com.

What do you think about Spirulina? Is it good for you?

I think so; I think it's is very good for health, and has lots nutrients, lots of vitamins, I don't specifically mention it here, but it is supposedly very packed with lots of good nutrients, so it is a good thing to add as a supplement or throw in a protein shake. A lot of the greens powders that I've used will have Spirulina as one of the ingredients in them. And you can get a lot of things in bars and shakes - whatever kind of form it comes in.

About fluoride; they put it in toothpaste – what you think of that?

Well, as much as we can minimize putting more fluoride in our systems we should, as well as maximizing the iodine to flush it out, but just as much we should also minimize putting more mercury and bromine in our bodies; we need to do the best we can at this.

How do you get good water?

Well, lots of people have different answers to that, I have a filter that I use here, and I have one at home. I used Nikken filters, but there are different water filters out there like Kangen Water Filters; there are a lot of companies that are probably pretty good, and I think that most of us should start with some kind of way to filter water.

If you do reverse osmosis, then make sure you're getting your minerals back in, whether through sea salts or through supplements; that's the way some people do it, you are also concerned about how is the pH going to be - not only is the water pure, but is the pH okay, can you add something in to balance the pH? Water is so good for us, yet you go to most stores, and it's all in plastic water bottles and it's been sitting out in the heat on a truck, filling it with more toxic chemicals, so it may be no better than tap water.

(Note: At this point a few other people brought up some things they learned about water that was interesting so we present it here. Research "Dr. Blaylock and distilled water," but for our purposes, we recommend pure water through filtering or reverse osmosis, and supplementing vitamins and minerals if needed.)

Speaker #1: And distilled water is not water you really want to drink because it is really mineral deficient, so you're actually going to find people who got sick from drinking distilled water. When it goes through the body, they talk about that water has a memory, and it binds to the minerals and leaches those minerals back out of the body, so distilled is definitely not a good choice if you're buying bottled water. You're better off buying spring water.

Speaker #2: Well do you remember Dr. Blaylock? He likes distilled water – it is in his newsletter. Well, maybe he put something back in the water too.

Dr. Culik: And of course he takes all kinds of minerals and supplements and stuff – maybe that's how he adjusts for that. And if you are not where you can get anything else, I guess that's an option, but if you can use some kind of good filter for your water, it is probably better.

(So there seems to be some controversy there. But at least consider using a filter, that's probably a good option here.)

BONUS: HEAVY METAL TOXICITIES, CHEMICALS AND BPA/PHTHALATES

(Note: This chapter is directly from our eBook called "The ABC Wellness Weightloss Pyramid.)

Chemicals and other toxins like heavy metals and BPA/Phthalates compose the last obstacle we will cover in our Weightloss Pyramid model. Again, so often people talk about chemical toxicities, heavy metals, pesticides, and phthalates as causing a problem or difficulty for those trying to lose weight.

TOXICITIES - SYMPTOMS
1) Fatigue and Chronic Fatigue Syndrome
2) Muscles Aches and Fibromyalgia
3) Difficult Weight Loss
4) Brain Fog
5) Fluid Retention
6) Low Thyroid
7) Numbness
8) Tremors, Restless Legs and Parkinson's

It has been reported that airline stewardesses, because of the chemicals sprayed in the cabins, the fire retardants, have a lot of chemical toxicities. But for the rest of us, there are certainly others who have exposures that may be harmful too. This includes people that might work in salons; persons doing hair and nails with toxic solutions, painters, and more. Definitely anyone who comes in with chronic fatigue and fibromyalgia, difficult weight loss, brain fog, fluid retention, low thyroid, and other issues like tremors, restless legs, and Parkinson's may have some contamination issues going on.

TOXICITIES - HISTORY
1) Prior or current Silver/Mercury amalgams
2) Prior or current Fish Intake esp. Tuna or Local
3) Prior or current Plastic Water Bottles
4) Prior or current Pesticides/Herbicides
5) Prior or current Tap water with Fluoride/Chlorine
6) Prior or current Bromine in Hot Tubs/Bromo-seltzer/Mountain Dew, Brominated (all) Flour
7) Prior or current flight in planes --- High Fire Retardant Sprays especially Pilots and Stewardesses

To address history of exposure, it may be silver fillings, fish intake, plastic water bottles, or pesticides. And you'd be amazed by how many people are spraying pesticides and chemicals in and around their house. Tap water can be toxic due to fluoride and chlorine, there is bromine in hot tubs and in airplanes the fire retardants may pose a problem. Try to be aware of what might be a toxin you need to avoid, and be careful when you have to use something potentially harmful.

TOXICITIES – EVALUATIONS
How do we evaluate people for toxicity? There are tests that can be done.

1) Urine Testing can be accurately done for heavy metals as long as a chelating chemical is used
2) Urine morning test for Phthalates and BPA
3) Testing is available for Pesticides

4) Testing can be done for other toxins

People can be urine tested with chelation to look for heavy metals, and there is a urine morning test for phthalates and BPA, and other tests exist for pesticides and other toxins. So, lots of companies have different specific tests and you should be able to find out more by researching the internet.

TOXICITIES – TREATMENTS

Here is a treatment list for exposure to toxic chemicals:

1) Identification leads to specific therapy for toxins....and helps avoid future exposures
2) Oral detoxification is possible with Zeolites, DMSA, Chlorella, Cilantro, EDTA-for metals
3) Detox pathways are improved with Methyl Folate, pure water, alkalinity
4) N-Acetyl Cysteine and Glutathione

As to treatment of toxicity, sometimes people say they just want to treat themselves and they can do oral detoxification with Zeolites, DMSA, Chlorella, Cilantro, and EDTA for metals, but whatever you do, please proceed cautiously and it is really recommended you consult with an experienced Health Practitioner who has dealt with numerous patients with the condition you suspect so you get an idea of how the detoxification process should normally proceed. This is especially helpful if you are not feeling well and do not know what to expect or how your body will react. Cleaning out the liver helps the body to detoxify and move the toxins out of the body and probiotics will help keep the bowels moving. But it is important to do it right, so expert help is always a great idea.

To continue with treatment of toxic chemicals, it is important to detox the liver phase 1 and 2 metabolism pathways. Here's what we recommend at ABC Wellness:

1) Dual-Tox from Numedica—includes Artichoke, ALA, NAC, MSM, Ellagic acid, Silymarin, Cal D Glucarate
2) Paleo Cleanse Shakes_from DFH with similar ingredients. Add to protein shakes or alone
3) ABC Wellness also uses Herbal Teas for Liver Detox and has a naturopath available for consultation

Some of the specific toxic chemical treatments I use include Dual-Tox from Numedica, which has many great ingredients in it. And there is a Paleo Cleanse Shake available that is a powder you can put in a protein shake or use alone - it is from Designs for Health (DFH) and has similar ingredients as Dual-Tox. Also, here at ABC Wellness, we have a Naturopath who has herbal teas for liver detox that she uses, so that is another option.

Here's more on treatment for chemical toxicities:

1) Amino acids, <u>minerals</u>, <u>vitamins</u> and <u>omega 3</u>s or <u>Krill oil</u> help--Glycine detoxes Phthalates and BPA
2) Paleo Cleanse from DFH: Powd-vit, min-Chrom/Vanadium, Aminos, Ca-D Glu, Taurine,

Silymarin,MSM, Inositol, Quercetin, Green Tea, NAC, Choline, Methionine, Dandelion, Glutathione
3) Good bowel function helps prevent reabsorption of toxins. Adequate magnesium, fiber and probiotics are part of the plan.
4) Cleanse drinks like herbal "Isa-Cleanse" from Isagenix removes toxins from fat.... to mobilize fat and fluids and maintain weight loss.

Again, when taking these supplements, make sure you're getting plenty of good amino acids, and Omega 3's. Paleo Cleanse has many helpful nutrients like Silymarin, green tea, and glutathione as well as many more. Also, make sure you are getting adequate amounts of magnesium, fiber and probiotics as this will help bowel function. Finally, ISA Cleanse is another product I've used over the years; it is from Isagenix and it helps clean the toxins out of the fat, and it helps to mobilize fats and fluids and to maintain weight loss.

What we covered should give you a good start on treating toxicities, but there may be other methods and supplements recommended by your own holistic practitioner. Whatever you do, proceed cautiously and safely, and research as much as you can about whatever methods you choose to use. If you experience discomfort when detoxing or cleansing, consult an expert you can trust on if it is OK to proceed.

If you liked this chapter and would like to learn more on the 9 obstacles, please use link below.

Lose Pounds Quickly by Overcoming Obstacles to Weightloss: **The eBook "<u>The ABC Wellness Weightloss Pyramid</u>" is live at Amazon and is available for purchase.**

Bonus – Smoothies for Weightloss and Superior Health

Smoothies are an excellent way to get vital nutrients in your daily diet, and if used with the proper ingredients and amounts, to lose pounds as well! Pick your favorite ingredients, and use the guidelines below to start. Modify recipes as you see fit, but try to do a bit of research on what items will best benefit you.

By concentrating on the elements you tend to lack in your daily diet, a daily smoothie may just be the answer you need to bring you up to maximum health and weightloss if desired. So, take the time to think about what might be the most beneficial smoothie you can make, and choose those ingredients to try. You can rotate with different recipes for variety as well in case you feel it's always the same old thing, and you want a new kind of taste.

Here is some basic guidance when preparing your smoothies.

Things to avoid:

Avoid NutraSweet and Splenda
Avoid Plastic water bottles for water source or drinking water
Avoid sugar, Agave and Honey if you are looking for weight loss.

Avoid Bananas--high glycemic and almost everyone I test is allergic and making antibodies to bananas
Avoid Dairy unless you have been tested for Casein and Whey and make no IgG Antibodies...a majority of patients I test are reactive to dairy and inflammation aggravates weight gain

Equipment Needed:

Use a Vitamix or Bullet or other powerful blender

Basic Items to Include:

Use a source of filtered water if available such as Nikken
Sweeteners - OK to use Stevia, Xylitol and/or B-Sweet from Boresha
Protein powder: Recommend Vegan from Numedica, Hemp powder, or Pea or Paleo from Designs for Health. The Paleo powder is sourced from Swedish cattle which are grass fed without pesticides and hormones. It is available in Vanilla or Chocolate.

Detoxification Nutrients You Can Add:

Paleo Cleanse Powder from Designs for Health
Raw sprouts, Ground flax seeds, Chia seeds
Radiant Greens powders from Tony O'Donnel, www.radiantgreens.com or Paleo Greens from Designs for Health, or Numedica Greens in Chocolate or Fruits and Greens in Strawberry-Kiwi flavors
Fruit Powders from Tony O'Donnel, or Designs for Health, or Numedica - also great options are Pomegranate powder, Blueberry powder, Acai powder, available from Amazon and others
Raw organic greens such as Kale and Spinach

Fresh or Frozen organic berries such as blueberry and raspberry
Fresh organic apples 1/2 to 1 added with skin.

Thickeners:

You can thicken with coconut milk, coconut half and half, coconut yogurt, coconut kefir. Use plain preferably without sweeteners. Before using almond or rice milk make sure you have IgG allergy testing since many people are allergic to these.
Oils such as 2 TBSP Coconut, or Flax Oil, or half an avocado
Bananas if not looking for weight loss.

More Flavor and Detoxification – try Essential Oils:

For detoxification and flavor you can add 1-2 drops of essential oils such as Lemon, Orange, Grapefruit, Lime from doTERRA which are safe and effective internally to help break down fat cells
Natural Oils such as Lemon and combinations like On Guard are fabulous for safe and very effective natural cleaning products to add to water and vinegar and avoid toxic chemical sprays and cleaners that can increase weight.
SLIM AND SASSY is an oil combination specifically meant to be added to water to help with weight loss by controlling appetite and dissolving fat cells.

Smoothie Recipes for Energy and Weight Loss

Lemon/Raspberry Smoothie

1 scoop Vanilla Pure Paleo Powder from Designs for Health
12 oz. pure water
1/2 cups raspberries fresh or frozen
2 drops Lemon Oil from doTERRA
1 Tablespoon Flax Oil
1 Tablespoon Ground Flax seed
1 scoop Paleo Cleanse powder from Designs for Health
1 scoop Paleo Greens from Designs for Health

Chocolate/Orange Smoothie

1 scoop Chocolate Pure Paleo Powder from DFH
1 scoop Paleo Cleanse Powder from DFH
1 scoop Radiant Greens from Tony O'Donnell
8 oz. coconut milk
1 Tbsp. Flax Oil
1 Tbsp. soaked Chia seeds
2 drops Wild Orange Essential Oil from doTERRA
4 oz. pure water

Fresh Lime Smoothie

1 scoop Numedica Vegan Vanilla Powder
8 oz. Almond Milk
1 scoop Numedica Power Greens
4 oz. pure water
1 Tbsp. Ground Flax Seed
1 Tbsp. MCT Oil
3 drops Lime Essential Oil from doTERRA

Optional Additions

For Leaky Gut: Glutamine Powder 1/2 - 1 tsp. at 2-4000 mg from Life Extension
For Joint Health: MSM Powder 1/2 tsp.
For Immunity: Vitamin C Powder-Buffered 2-4000mg from Life Extension

For Immunity and Sugar: Bitter Melon powder 1 tsp.
For constipation, headaches, muscles cramps: Magnesium chelate powder available from Prothera etc
For Detox and Fluid Retention: Add Cleanse for Life Powder from Isagenix
Extra Nutrients: Organic Raw Spinach, Kale, Apple, Berries
Note: Many people are allergic to Bananas and also Strawberry is a frequent allergen so I usually avoid them

References:

For **doTERRA Oils**, go to: http://www.mydoterra.com/abcwellness/

For **Numedica products**, go to: www.drculik.com and look for NUTRITION across the top - you can search for the following terms on the site to see helpful, related products: Adrenal Support, Thyroid Support, Detoxification, Gluten Sensitivity and Metabolic Management for supplement support.

For **Designs for Health**, as well as **Prothera Probiotics**, B12/Folate and more, go to: www.dssorders.com/abcwellness and use access code "dc374" to order - you can search PALEO for shakes and greens powders etc.

For **Pure Encapsulations** supplements and vitamins go to: www.purecapspro.com/drculik - go to ALL DEPARTMENTS and scroll to WEIGHT LOSS SUPPORTS (Options include: Chromium, Cinnamon,

ABC Wellness "Simple Steps to Better Health!"

CLA, Pure Clear Powder, Pure Lean Nutrients, Pure Green Coffee Packets and more)

Thank-you again for joining us and good luck on your journey to a healthier, you!

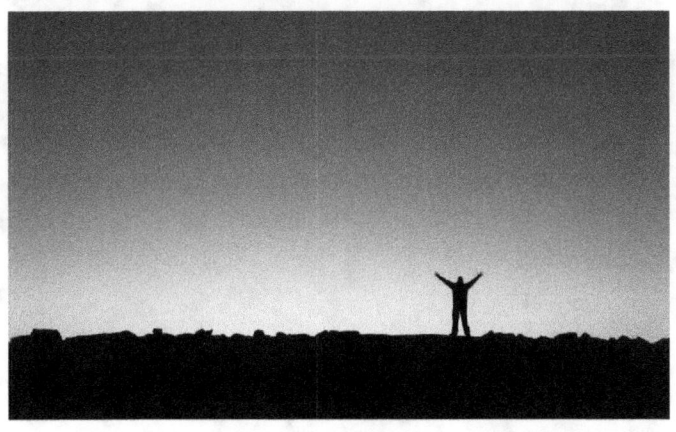

BONUS: ESSENTIAL OILS FOR HEALTH AND LONGEVITY

How would you like to upgrade your healthcare today naturally, without expensive medications and doctor's visits, saving you time, money and decreasing stress and aggravation? Is this even possible? Could it really be true? The answer is now a resounding yes, and it comes through the use of Essential Oils. Essential Oils are a hot topic these days, and becoming more popular as people realize the benefit of using them to stay healthy.

They come from the heart of plants and are considered "Nature's Medicine Cabinet". But please remember that the quality and purity of these Essential Oils are vital to a positive experience, so try to find ones of high quality. Your body deserves the best, so choose wisely.

The ones that I use and represent are called doTerra. Only doTerra offers Certified Pure Therapeutic Grade (CPTG) Essential Oils and Supplements. They are Certified Pure Pharmaceutical Grade (CPTG) and many of them can be inhaled as vapors or applied topically on the body, especially on the feet. They also can be taken internally by mixing with water or putting them into capsules. Here is more information on how I personally use these essential oils, but certainly, you may find your own favorite ways to apply them.

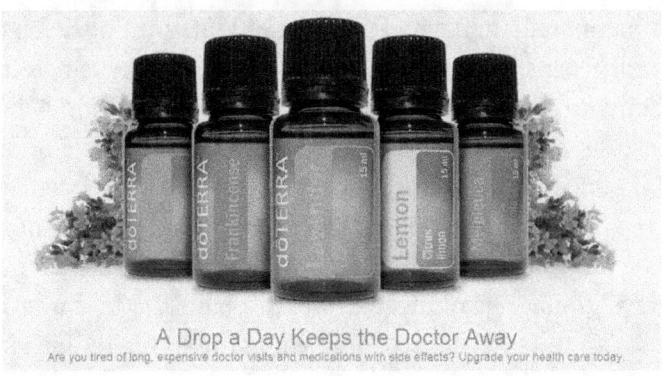

A Drop a Day Keeps the Doctor Away

Are you tired of long, expensive doctor visits and medications with side effects? Upgrade your health care today.

OnGuard is one of my favorites and is a combination of Wild Orange, Clove, Cinnamon, Eucalyptus and Rosemary. I carry a small bottle of "beadlets" in my purse and pop 2 or 3 in my mouth to freshen breath or at the first sign of any throat irritation. The outer cover dissolves and gives a fresh blast of cleansing oils. I also use the pure oil to put drops into a capsule every day along with other oils, I usually use 3-5 drops of OnGuard as a general preventive for infection and inflammation. Keeping infections at bay naturally and safely is reassuring and good for the body.

Toothpaste: I use the **Onguard** Toothpaste and it is amazingly cleansing for the mouth and it tastes great.

Counter, Hand and Laundry Cleanser: A few drops of **Onguard** oil in water in a spray bottle clean my counters and I put it in my detergent to clean and freshen laundry; I also use the foaming hand soap in the bathroom.

Frankincense is another oil I have come to appreciate and love. The herb Frankincense has been documented and used since 1500 BC by physicians and priests. It has been called LIQUID GOLD since it helps so many conditions from mood to acne and skin lesions and studies have shown it even has benefits for cancer. The gum resin is extracted from Boswellia trees in Oman for the doTERRA oils. Frankincense has been and still is a major trading commodity. In ancient days, tons of frankincense was transported by camels port to port because people valued it so highly for its amazing benefits.

General Wellbeing: I use 1-2 drops of **Frankincense** every morning on each of my feet after my bath and let the oils absorb in well through the larger pores. I also add 3-5 drops to my daily capsule of oil with **Onguard**.

Candida Suppression: I usually add 2-3 drops of **Oregano** to my oral capsule for suppressing yeast.

Drinking Water or Tea: I use 2-3 drops of **Lemon, Lime or Slim and Sassy** oil in my water or tea.

Facial Cleansing: I add 1 drop of **Lemon** into soapy hands before I scrub my face to dissolve oils and grime from the skin and pores. I usually add it to **Onguard** for cleaning sprays.

Sinus Congestion and Allergies: I inhale a few drops of **Peppermint** after rubbing them in my palms for alertness and opening up the sinuses for congestion or allergies.

Sleep and Relaxation: For sleep and calming at night I use **<u>Lavender</u>** on my feet, pillow and rub in palms and inhale.

Pet Use: I also use **<u>Lavender</u>** on the pads of my dog's feet for calming effect. **Sprains, Sore Muscles, and Headaches**: **<u>Deep Blue</u>** is an oil for topical use only and also comes as a cream. I have used it for sprained ankles, sore muscles and on the temples for headaches. It has fabulous properties for discomfort and inflammation.

For even more information, you can check out the extensive benefits and uses of OnGuard and Frankincense and any other oils of interest at www.everythingessential.me. You can also look up symptoms or conditions and see recommended oils.

If interested, ABC Wellness carries these oils at: www.mydoterra.com/abcwellness.

BONUS: PAW PAW EXTRACT – A SUPPLEMENT TO HELP YOU LIVE TO 100

Fabulous Nutrients from Nature's Sunshine: Have you heard about the Paw Paw? Strange name, yes, but it just might be a supplement you can use occasionally in your quest to live to the ripe old age of 100. Paw Paw tastes like a cross between a banana and a mango and Paw Paw trees grow in 26 states in the United States, growing wild from the Gulf Coast up to the Great Lakes region.

The Paw Paw fruit has yellow-green skin and soft, orange flesh which has earned it the nickname "custard apple," but it also goes by "poor man's banana" and "Indiana banana." This fruit has a creamy, custard-like consistency and a delicious, sweet flavor. Here is a picture, and you can google "Paw Paw" for more information.

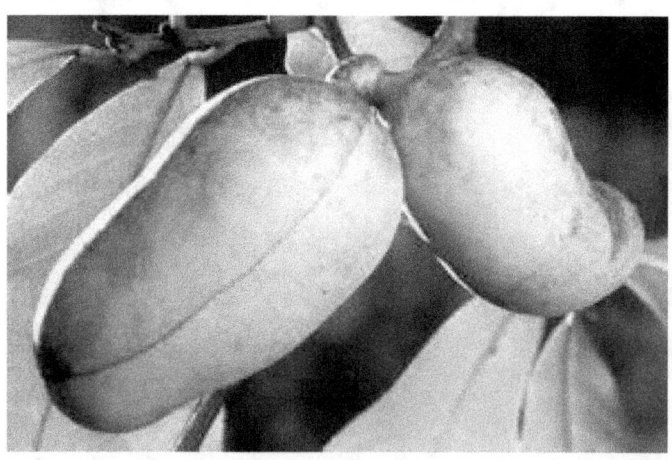

Paw Paw Cell-Reg by Nature's Sunshine: Now if you can find the fruit locally, you can enjoy it as a that way, but if not, you do have the option to take advantage of its benefits by taking capsules that contain an extract from the Paw Paw tree's twigs.

Benefits of Paw Paw:

1. Supports the immune system.
2. Selectively affects specific cells.
3. Modulates ATP production in specific cells.
5. Modulates blood supply to specific cells.

How Paw Paw Works:

The active compounds in Paw Paw Cell-Reg are a mixture of over 50 acetogenins. Acetogenins are active compounds that affect the production of ATP (Adenosine Triphosphate) in the mitochondria (the powerhouse) of the cell. ATP is the cells' major source of energy. Acetogenins selectively modulate the production of ATP in specific cells. Modulating the production of ATP affects the viability of specific cells and may help modulate the blood supply to them. Acetogenins also support and enhance the effectiveness of conventional medical regimens.

A clinical study with over 100 participants showed that the Paw Paw extract, containing a mixture of acetogenins, supports the body's normal cells during times of cellular stress. Paw Paw Cell-Reg is the only standardized acetogenin product available to regulate specific cells. Nature's Sunshine uses an extract of the twigs of the North American Paw Paw tree, which contain the most concentrated amount of acetogenins. These twigs are harvested when they are most biologically active, and the extract is standardized biologically using an invertebrate bioassay. This is a renewable resource since the tree is not harmed during the harvest.

Ingredients: Paw Paw twig extract.

Recommended Use: Take 2 capsules with food three times daily. Do not exceed recommended serving size or nausea may occur.

NOTE: Co-Q10, Thyroid Support and 7-Keto may decrease the effectiveness of this product. Only those with cellular abnormalities should take this product on a regular/daily basis. Do not take this product if you are pregnant, think you may become pregnant, or if you are breastfeeding.

How to Obtain Paw Paw Capsules: Go to www.naturessunshine.com Search Paw Paw. At check-out you can either pay retail or join the company and get the Wholesale price. If you prefer the wholesale discount, please join under Dr. Culik.

The ID to join under Dr. Culik is 3232529

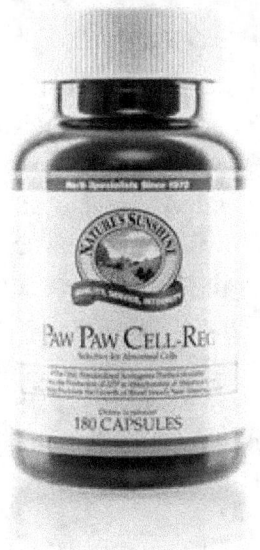

BONUS: DIET AND EXERCISE

At this point, you want to focus on diet and exercise and you can follow your favorite program if you have one, but for those who don't I have supplied references for both diet and exercise, and you are free to investigate and follow any of these as I recommend them highly. We will also recommend another program at the end if you want more of a coaching program. Whatever plan you choose, I would suggest you follow just one plan at a time; using elements of other plans is OK though if the plan you are following provides no guidance.

BASIC NUTRITIONAL PLAN RECOMMENDED

After all the evaluations, we now move on to diet and exercise. First, we will start with a basic nutritional plan for you to follow unless you have received other guidance from a qualified expert:

1) Lots of purified water
2) Protein Breakfast within 1 hour of awakening
3) Protein at every meal
4) Protein Shake at least 1/day per food sensitivities
5) Greens and Fruits Powders- for nutrients and alkalinity
6) Avoid Simple carbs: bread, rice, potatoes, pasta
7) No sugar even natural: Ok <u>B-Sweet</u> or Xylitol
8) Low glycemic veggies 3-6 per day

The beauty of the ABC Wellness Weightloss Pyramid method is it allows you to adopt any other methods you wish to try as far as diet and exercise – this plan is going to make all those other methods work better and faster because it is about eliminating problem areas that once held you back. But for those without a specific plan to follow, what comes next here is basic information gained from various experts and this should serve you well if you just want to follow this advice!

First, I just listed out a quick nutritional plan that includes lots of pure water, a protein breakfast within one hour of awakening, it may be a protein shake (have one shake per day), protein in every meal, greens or fruit powders, which are great for energy, avoiding the simple carbs like bread, rice, potatoes, pasta, and using either no sugar, or a healthy, safe sweetener like Boresha's B-Sweet or xylitol, and lots of low glycemic veggies 3-6 times per day.

DIET PLANS AVAILABLE

Here are some diet references for your convenience. These are healthy, low carb and Paleo type diets that can really make a difference for you!

1) **www.thepaleodiet.com Dr. Loren Cordain***
2) **www.jonnybowden.com Weight Loss Plans***
3) **www.theprimalblueprint.com web site and book**
4) **www.marksdailyapple.com free primal recipes**
5) **www.drhyman.com The Blood Sugar Solution Book and Cookbook**
6) **www.tanaamen.com The Omni Diet Book, wife of Dr. Daniel Amen Tana is an RN and fitness expert**

7) Also: We have a Registered Dietician and Weight Loss Expert Available at ABC Wellness...

See if any of these make sense for your particular situation. We recommend a low-carb diet, like a Paleo Diet, and there are several references here like Jonny Bowden, Primal Blue Print, and Dr. Hyman, who has a lot of information on sugar and the low glycemic diet, and there is a new book out called the Omni Diet by Dr. Tana's wife. For those interested and those in the local area, ABC Wellness has a dietitian here who does take individual patients and discusses nutrients and a diet specifically for them.

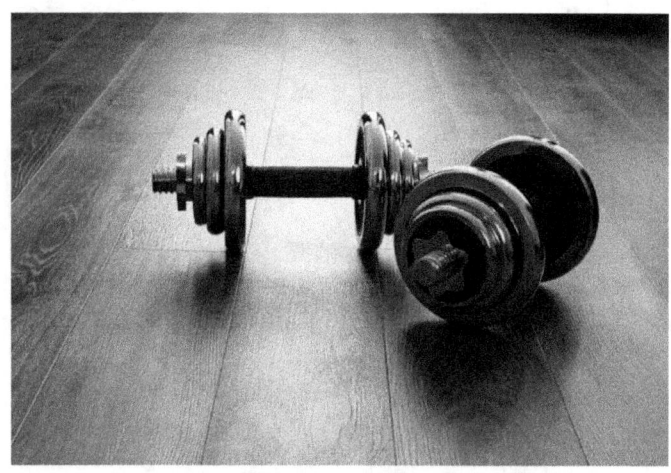

EXERCISE PLANS

1) Aerobic Exercise: Walk, Treadmill, Swim, Bike
2) Muscle building Anaerobic: Weights/Resistance
3) www.alsearsmd.com Dr. Al Sears PACE plan
4) Not monotonous cardio exercises but quick 10 minute routines with variable Pace.
5) Start a time, place, partner and put it on your schedule. At least 3 times a week and increase time and intensity.

About exercise plans, you are pretty much free to devise your own program, or use your favorite trainer's routine although we will make one recommendation to think about.

To start out, whether it is for five minutes or half an hour, just get yourself moving! You can begin with walking, using a treadmill, swimming, biking, or even doing some muscle building and weights, but start slow and easy and build up gradually whatever you decide to do. There is no use going overboard like some folks do when they first start a new routine. An injury to yourself will just set you back and is not worth it.

That said, you may want to consider the PACE plan as referenced. I love this book, and Dr. Al Sears is a doctor that recommends quick, maximum energy outputs, and to do short routines instead of the general walking or aerobics for five hours. He says you can get the energy and build it up fast and more naturally when you do like our ancestors did, kind of like the Paleo diet, but this is Paleo Exercise!

Thyroid Adrenal Secrets Revealed

You know, our ancestors might chase that wild animal for 10 minutes, and then walk. And they probably weren't jogging for hours or days, just a short amount of time. So consider using this kind of routine – it might be easier to stick on this kind of routine long term, which is crucial for long term results and keeping the weight off.

FINAL SPECIAL BONUS: 25 STEP HEALING PROGRAM EBOOK

We are including the entire 25 Step Healing Program as a free gift to you in this release! It starts on the next page...this is a special test release to see if it is appreciated. If you do appreciate the extra book as a bonus, please consider leaving a positive review on Amazon because we noticed books need this attention to get people to try them. Thank-you!

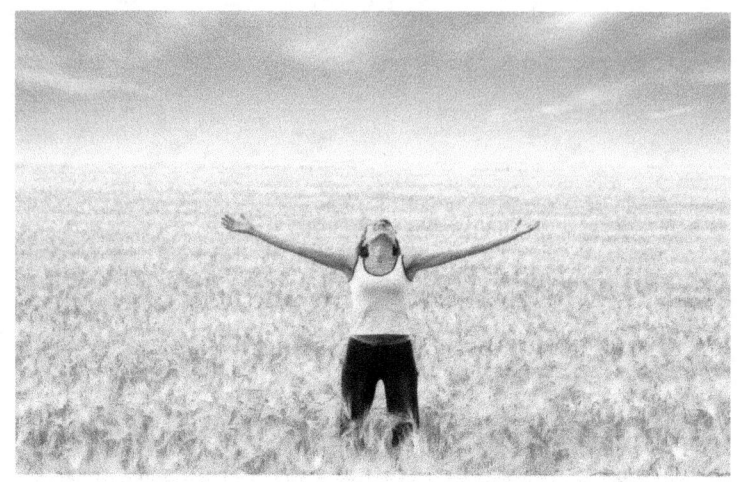

25 STEP
HEALING
PROGRAM

A SHORT SELF-HELP GUIDE TO HEALING THROUGH
HEALTH ASSESSMENT, EVALUATION AND TESTING,
PHYSICAL EXAMINATION AND PRUDENT ACTIONS
TO AID YOUR THYROID, ADRENALS & WHOLE BODY

DIANE CULIK, MD

25 Step
Healing
Program!

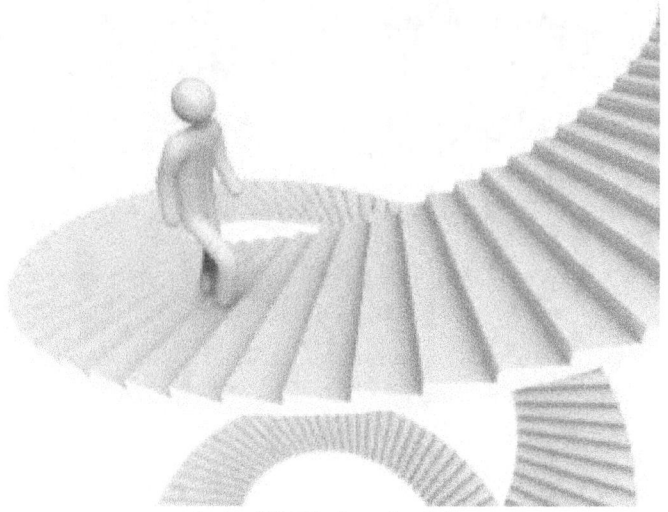

A Self-Help Guide

Attention: If you feel tired, frazzled, maybe just a bit worn down, or you just want a guide to give you some natural, alternative, yet practical health tips and tricks leading to feeling super, this may be the guide you are looking for. It concentrates on things that Dr. Culik has found to be helpful for most people. Don't miss out – this information might change your life!

25 Step Healing Program:

A Short Self-Help Guide to Healing though Health Assessment, Evaluation and Testing, Physical Examination and Prudent Actions To Aid Your Thyroid, Adrenals and Whole Body

Diane Culik, MD
Kyle Weed

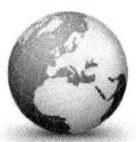

ABW111
ABW111 Publishing, Inc.
A Better World Company

ABC Wellness "Simple Steps to Better Health!"

Limits of Liability/Disclaimer of Warranty

Disclaimer: This information is for educational purposes only, and not meant to substitute for medical attention. If you have concerns with anything you want to try as a result of your learning here, please see your primary physician.

The authors and publishers of this book have used their best efforts in preparing this program. The author and publishers of this book make no representation or warranties with respect to the accuracy, applicability, fitness, or completeness of the contents of this program. They disclaim any warranties, express or implied, of merchantability or fitness for any particular purpose. The authors and publisher shall in no event be held liable for any loss or other damage, including but not limited to special, incidental, consequential, or other damages. The authors and publisher do not warrant performance, effectiveness, or applicability of any sites listed in this book. All links are for information purposes only and are not warranted for content, accuracy or any other implied or explicit purpose.

This manual contains material protected under international and federal copy right laws and treaties. Any unauthorized reprint or use of this material is prohibited.

Introduction

What is this book about?

This eBook provides a roadmap to improving your health in general, and thyroid adrenal health specifically. It contains 25 immediate steps anyone can take which may help them determine what is going on with their body, and take actions to fix it. The result may be to help you lose weight, have more energy, and just plain feel better than they do now.

Please note that this is not a long, theoretical book. It is not meant to be – it is meant to provide immediate action steps to get to the source of your health issues, so please, if you can afford it, do the testing and find out what the results say. Then take action based on your interpretation of those results. You can use the table of contents as a checklist and proceed through each item! And use your instincts or internal "hunches" as to what might be affecting you.

In other words, focus in on those areas you feel guided to – where you feel something might be going on and further investigation is merited. Your own wisdom can really help guide you to some meaningful answers many times, when an outsider would really have no idea without running multiple tests, and tests will often not reveal the truth completely. Think about your lifestyle, your habits, and your environment – could there be anything having an effect on you that you perhaps assumed was insignificant?

Be willing to experiment for a few days with a new way of doing things if you can – maybe what you discover will shed new light on what is going on. But one thing has become clearer and clearer over the years – many of us have been underactive physically, eating the Standard American Diet of refined and processed foods, and living with toxic exposures that really are not good for us – or our thyroid and adrenal glands.

(Helpful Tip: If you are reading this book, we believe you are probably beyond the basics as far as knowing what thyroid and adrenal glands are and how they work. However, as a refresher, and for some great information and explanations of how these glands work and what they do, please google "Thyroid" and/or "Adrenal" Glands, and check out some of the better sites with pictures like Web MD or Wikipedia.)

Why write a book about healing in 25 steps and focusing on thyroid and adrenals?

Are you perhaps not feeling as well as you might feel at your healthiest? Are you in shape, and at your ideal weight? This book might help, and that is why it is being written – to give you a set of ACTIONs you can take to not only find out what is wrong, but even take some steps to immediately correct any imbalance.

ABC Wellness "Simple Steps to Better Health!"

Over time certain patterns of illnesses appear in our population, and it seems many people go through similar types of problems. Over time, patterns emerge, and certain tests prove useful in diagnosing what is going on with these people and certain actions become the go-to activities needed to address these illnesses. Follow these steps, and it is very likely you will find some things you can do better on.

At the end, forgive us the sales pitches for the other books, but some of these might have some other advice you might want to consider – like how to live to 100, or how to heal your whole body. We truly hope you do not feel the price is too high for these books, which are all under $10. After all, what does one trip to the doctor cost you today? Think on this – this advice could serve you for many years to come. What is that worth? You will spend more on a fast food lunch than this! Anyway, to continue....

At this time, there appears to be an epidemic of people walking around with thyroid issues and probably adrenal issues as well. It is estimated there are over 59 million people who may be experiencing some kind of thyroid problem, and most of them don't have a clue that this may be happening. Why? A couple of reasons seem apparent.

First, the soil is depleted of many minerals, including iodine, and iodine is critical for the thyroid to function. So the food you get in your grocery store in many cases does not contain sufficient nutrition to fuel the body properly. Recent tests in Michigan showed that over 95% of participants were low in iodine, so it's very possible that you are also.

Second, there are many toxins in the environment and in our food supply that affect us and our thyroid and adrenal glands and interfere with the functioning of these systems. It is important that you know what some of these toxins are so you can reduce or eliminate them from your life. We will cover more on both these issues later in this e-book, but suffice it to say that you are doing yourself a great favor by learning what the truth might be here.

Why is this important to you? What can you gain from knowing this? A lot - the benefits are myriad...

1. First, your health will be greatly improved by eliminating toxins and improving your diet and by ensuring you get adequate amounts of iodine and other critical nutrients. We will go over some of these items in this e-book.
2. Second, if you are overweight, the poor functioning of your thyroid may be the primary obstacle to why you cannot lose weight, and addressing this issue may mean major success.
3. Third, getting your thyroid and adrenals into proper shape will mean a less stressed out you. You will be able handles issues and challenges in your life a lot better when you have balanced your thyroid and adrenal glands.

4. Fourth, there is a lot of confusion about proper testing of thyroid and adrenals, and we will cover that also.

5. Fifth, following the advice we give may allow you to straighten out problem areas, and get into the best shape of your life through proper exercise and diet.

About the Authors - who are we and why should you listen to us?

This book is a collaboration between Diane Culik, MD, and Kyle Weed, independent health researcher. When two people work together, the end result of their efforts is often synergistic, and much more benefit is derived by the end consumer. What follows below is a write-up for each of us, and then a short explanation as to why we working together will benefit you as someone wishing to improve their health.

Dr. Diane Culik, MD, brings you natural health solutions, and is a top thyroid-adrenal doctor with over 30 years' experience! After graduating from the University of Michigan Medical School, Dr. Culik began practicing medicine a number of years ago, following the traditional path, learning the best that conventional medicine had to offer. About 17 years ago, she switched to Holistic Medicine, and now blends the two approaches so you get the best of both worlds! She recently opened ABC Wellness, which stands for Alternative-Balanced-Comprehensive, in Sterling Heights, Michigan where she offers all patients "Simple Steps to Better Health." Her goal is to assist you in finding the path to a better way of life through the removal of obstacles to healing like environmental toxins and nutritional deficiencies and allowing the body to heal itself.

Kyle Weed is an independent health researcher, a writer, and communicator, with a "Vision" of reaching people through a variety of media and creating happiness, healing, and peace. He currently works with ABC Wellness to create eBooks, and DVD/Video Programs on Natural Health Topics such as anti-aging, cancer survival secrets, thyroid and adrenal care, weightloss, and more. Kyle felt led to this experience through inner guidance after years of suffering through mercury toxicity caused in part by "silver" fillings, and after extensively researching the health field, reading through hundreds of health and medical books, websites and other literature. His goal is to bring Alternative Health Secrets, both ancient and new and unique Healing Modalities, Forgiveness and Mind Training Techniques and any other helpful healing information to public awareness.

How do the two of us working together offer a greater benefit to you, the reader, and user of possible life changing alternative health secrets?

By working together, the two of us fill in gaps each one of us working and writing independently may have missed. Dr. Culik provides the credibility of a trained medical doctor, can offer authoritative knowledge on many topics, and also the safety factor only a trained medical professional can offer, while still retaining a mind open to new and unusual alternative healing techniques. She will be the one providing the step by step instructions for this eBook based on her experience with patients, and her knowledge of thyroid and adrenal issues.

Kyle Weed, having undergone a lengthy health challenge and an equally lengthy period of studying health techniques and information can often definitively state in many cases what really worked to bring healing and comfort to himself and others undergoing similar experiences. As I (Kyle Weed) am the one pulling the information together, and adding to it, I can state that I have personally read and studied tons of material from the leading alternative, natural doctors on the scene today, so both Dr. Culik and I will bring you the best of the best in alternative health care, including top secrets you can use right now!

Disclaimer: Of course, we have to state that this information is for educational purposes only, and not meant to substitute for medical attention. If you have concerns with anything you want to try as a result of your learning here, please see your primary physician. Most things we mention are proven to be safe - foods, supplements, and testing methods you can try at home inexpensively, but please do err on the side of caution when trying anything. Start with small doses or trials and work up gradually if possible. This is especially the case when detoxifying the body. We provide more free information if you sign up at http://thyroid-adrenal-solutions.com, but we also recommend you work with a holistic practitioner who understands how to safely proceed.

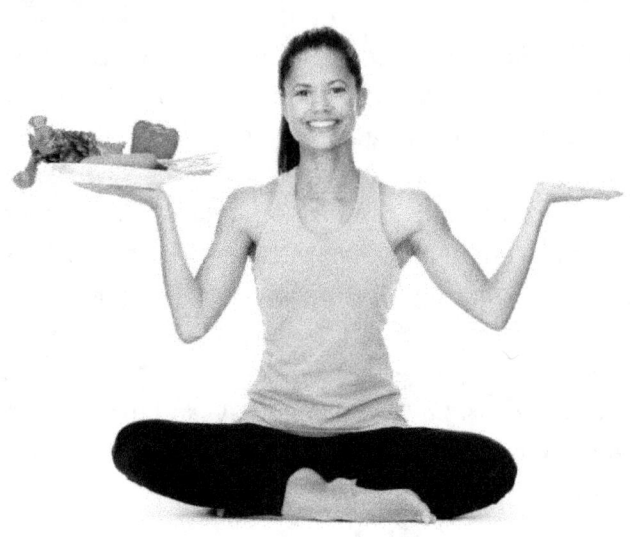

Steps 1 – 5, Complete Lab Testing for Thyroid, Complete Physical Exam for Thyroid, Thyroid Questionnaire, Morning Body Temperature Test, and Food Allergy Testing.

Hi, I'm Diane Culik, and I would like to talk to you today about Thyroid Disease, and specifically "Is your thyroid disease being missed or mistreated?"

I want to go through 25 different things and steps or ways to improve your thyroid and adrenals that you need to know about to properly evaluate, treat, and improve your thyroid and adrenal glands. Are you afflicted with a thyroid issue? Follow steps 1-5 and find out for sure. If you are, you can start taking action to feel better immediately!

(Note: At the beginning of this manual there are a few questions that we had originally gathered some information from the internet in order to help answer the question. We have since removed that material as to not infringe on any copyrights. However, we will inform you to Google a certain subject, and you can read up on some great information and instructions to supplement what Dr. Culik has presented. Sorry for any inconvenience, but we strive to do things correctly.)

1. Complete Lab Testing for the Thyroid (Free T3, Free T4, TSH, TPO, ATG, Reverse T3)

ONE, you need complete thyroid blood testing. A TSH test alone is not adequate to decide if you have thyroid disease. You really must know not only your free T3, free T4, TSH, your thyroid antibodies, which include TPO and ATG, but you have to know your Reverse T3 to see if you have inactive thyroid production. Anyone of those may be enough to indicate that you have thyroid disease. So if you don't have the whole panel, your physician isn't doing enough to evaluate your thyroid. (Google: Complete Thyroid Lab Testing)

2. Complete Physical Exam for Thyroid conditions: Skin, Hair, Nails, Eyebrows, Thyroid Gland, Pretibial Edema, Reflexes

Number TWO, you need a complete exam for your thyroid. Thyroid Disease can be picked up on your blood work, but also many findings from your physical exam will suggest if you have thyroid problems.

You have to examine the skin for dryness, flakiness, and itching, and see if the hair is thinning. Nails can be pitted, and lateral brow thinning is a common problem; the thyroid gland itself can show nodularity or enlargement. Sometimes this is subtle, sometimes very severe. Pretibial edema can be obvious, or just some mild pitting or denting of the legs when you press on them with your thumb may be a finding. Also the reflexes of the lower extremities can be an indication of thyroid problems. (Google: Thyroid, Physical Exam)

3. Review and complete Thyroid Questionnaire of Symptoms: This would be helpful to take to an open minded Doctor

We have a complete thyroid questionnaire, number THREE, which may be a significant help in indicating if you have thyroid problems. You really need to go through this one by one, check off the items that seem relevant to you, and take this to an open minded physician, who can evaluate all your symptoms. A great place to start is to go to www.acam.org for Holistic Physicians. We have looked at your labs, your physical findings, and now your symptoms all by themselves may be a strong indicator of thyroid problems.

Thyroid Quiz and Symptom Evaluation (check any positives)

(____) Sensitivity to cold or Hands and feet are usually cold

(____) Morning temperatures are less than 97.8

(____) Wear socks to bed often

(____) Dry or scaly skin

(____) Need to apply lotion and oils frequently

(____) Often daily fatigue

(____) Never seem to get enough sleep or naps for energy

(____) Memory and concentration are decreased

(____) Hair is thinning, course, dry, breaking off

(____) Nails are thin, chip, peal or break

(____) Lower legs are puffy, or indent with pressure

(____) Hands and fingers are puffy

(____) Carpel Tunnel symptoms

(____) Outer third of eyebrows are thin or absent

(____) Libido or sex drive has decreased or is low

(____) Weight is difficult to lose or gain even when dieting

(____) Bowels are sluggish or constipated or need to take laxatives

(____) Autoimmune diseases like Rheumatoid, Lupus, and Vitiligo

(____) Low B12 or Pernicious Anemia

(____) Known or suspected food allergies or Celiac disease

(____)   Silver Amalgams now or in the past (Mercury fillings)

(____)   History of radiation therapy to neck or chest

(____) Drinking now or prior, water with chlorine and/or fluoride

(____) Eat moderate amounts of Soy milk, cheese, burgers, dressings, oil etc

(____)   Family History of any type of Thyroid Problems

(____)   Eat fish frequently esp. tuna, sushi, non-wild Salmon

(____) Moody, depressed, irritable, apathetic

4. Measure your morning body temperature (ok over 97.8). Document for several days and for women before ovulation

Number FOUR, your body temperature is very important in evaluating if you have thyroid concerns, since the thyroid gland sets the metabolic rate. To check your thyroid, you can evaluate how your morning temperature is compared to normal, which should be 98.6, or maybe minus a degree. If it is less than 97.6, than you really have possible thyroid issues. Many people run 95 or 96 and their doctors tell them, "that's just the way you are, your temperature runs low." But usually there is a reason for it and most often it's because your thyroid isn't completely functioning. (Google: Basal Body Temperature Measurement)

5. Food Allergy testing if any thyroid antibodies or symptoms, especially IgG or IgA Antibodies for gluten and casein

Number FIVE, is food allergy testing. This is something critical if there is any concern with thyroid disease and especially if you have elevated thyroid antibodies. Food allergies are so common today that probably everyone should have them done. And this has to be blood work with IGG or IGA blood tests. The skin test or IGE blood tests that an allergist or a pulmonary specialist might do are going to have nothing to do with whether your food allergies are significant related to your thyroid. Those are going to be related to peanut allergy or asthma problems. But you have to specifically ask for and get IGG or IGA blood tests, especially for gluten, which is related to wheat; and casein, which is a protein in dairy. (Google: Food Allergy Testing)

STEPS 6 – 10, NUTRITIONAL CONSULTATION, HEAVY METAL TESTING, VITAMIN TESTING, SPECTRACELL TESTING AND THYROID TOXINS TO AVOID

6. Nutritionist Consultation if Food Allergies are documented to ensure avoidance of foods that are often a risk

Number SIX, if you have any food allergy findings, anything positive, you really should see a nutritionist, and especially a holistic nutritionist to help you review what you are eating, what you can change, and how you can revise your diet. If there are several food allergies that are elevated, you may want to consider a complete blood panel of IGG blood testing, and several of the laboratories like Bio Tek are able to do that from even just a little finger stick of blood.

7. Heavy Metal testing if Amalgams, Fish intake, or other exposures or neurologic symptoms such as tremor/ numb/ brain fog

Number SEVEN, heavy metal testing should definitely be done if you have any amalgams or silver fillings, if you eat or ever ate any significant amount of fish, certainly if you have exposures, just being near a coal factory that is coal burning. Also certainly be tested if

163

you have any neurological symptoms, any tremor, any symptoms of Parkinson's, multiple sclerosis, any brain fog, chronic fatigue, fibromyalgia; all of these can be related to heavy metal toxicity.

8. Vitamin testing for Zinc, Selenium, B Vitamins, etc.

Number EIGHT, vitamin testing is very essential, and the things that are most related to thyroid problems are zinc levels, and especially red blood cell zinc level is important, your serum selenium is significant; those are both required for thyroid conversion in the cells to the active form (T4 to T3 conversion). And B vitamins are also essential, especially to measure B1, B6, and B12.

9. Spectracell Testing for Intracellular Nutrient Levels. Measure 33 including Vitamin C, K, E, Bs, Biotin, CoQ10, ALA, Selenium, Chromium, Calcium/Magnesium/Zinc/ Copper, Glutathione, Inositol, Carnitine, Serine, Glutamine etc.

Number NINE, for more complete testing, there are labs such as Spectra-Cell that can do a very comprehensive analysis of intracellular nutrients, and they will measure 33 different vitamins, many that you can't get from a regular lab such as vitamin C, vitamin K, vitamin E, certainly all the B vitamins, but also Biotin, CoQ10, Alpha-Lipoic Acid, selenium, chromium, calcium, which is the only way to get an accurate level, not possible from traditional labs, magnesium, zinc, copper, glutathione, Carnitine, serine, glutamine, on and on. So this is a very helpful test, and everyone I have tested so far has one, and usually several deficiencies that are essential to correct for maximizing your health.

10. Avoid Soy, Fluoride, Bromine, Chlorine, PFOAs, Teflon

Number TEN, definitely avoid the toxic things that interfere with the thyroid and these absolutely are Soy, Fluoride, Bromine, Chlorine, PFOAs and Teflon. Soy, of course you know if you use Soy Milk or eat Soy Beans, but Soy is hidden in many foods, such as dressings and processed foods. Fluoride, of course you are probably going to have in your water, your shower, fluoride added toothpaste and mouthwash, so you want to get natural sources and filter your water. Bromine is very toxic. Bromo-Seltzer, brominated hot tubs, pretty much any processed flour now has bromine in it. And Chlorine is also in our tap water, great to kill off the bacteria, but damages the good bacteria in our gut and interferes with iodine. Teflon and PFOAs are also toxic and interfere with our thyroid. These are usually going to be in either plastic bottles or coated pans.

Steps 11 – 15, More Thyroid Toxins to Avoid, Adequate Sleep, Vital Supplements for Thyroid and Adrenals Including Vitamin C and Unprocessed Sea Salt, Liver Detoxification

11. Avoid Mercury Amalgams, Toxic Vaccinations (Flu Shots) and Fish (OK Pacific Wild Salmon)

Continuing with more items to help your thyroid, Number ELEVEN is absolutely avoid any mercury amalgams, silver fillings have 50% mercury in them, also flu shots have, still, mercury in them, even though many vaccines have taken them out, and they put this in the vaccines they give adults as well as pregnant women and children. It's not good for your thyroid. Fish, basically limit to Wild Pacific Salmon, all other fish are going to have mercury in them and not worth the risk.

12. Adequate Sleep: use Melatonin (3-20 mg) or Herbal Teas such as Valerian/ Chamomile as needed or GABA

Number TWELVE; you really need adequate sleep to support both your thyroid and adrenals. Very good for improving sleep is melatonin; you can start at 3 mg and you can double and triple the dose. It's very safe, and for people with immune deficiencies, or cancer, even 20 or 40 mg can be used. For other options, you can use herbal teas, chamomile, valerian, hops are very helpful, and GABA can be obtained in capsules, or now we even have the chewable GABA that not only helps sleep, but for anxiety and stress disorders.

13. Adequate Vitamin C 2-4,000mg /day is reasonable, more for Adrenal or Chronic Fatigue

Number THIRTEEN, vitamin C is good for every human being on the planet, and it's really critical for fatigue and especially for adrenal fatigue and adrenal burnout. Vitamin C is not made by human beings or other primates, also fruit bats and guinea pigs are not able to make vitamin C in their liver, we lost the ability, so we need to take in more vitamin C than just what is needed to prevent scurvy and die within a few months. We need it for our vascular system, our joints, our connective tissue, and absolutely for our adrenals – at least 2000 mg a day, is the preferred dose. It is available from Life Extension, from Pure Encapsulations, and you can get it in capsules, sometimes powdered, buffered form, and even chewable. It's excellent for kids to adults, any age. For adults at least 2000 mg, children, 1000 mg would be reasonable.

14. Use unprocessed sea salt for adrenals (only Non White is Right—pink, grey or beige)

Next, number FOURTEEN, salt is very important for the body. Our bodies require salt, and you need to use unprocessed sea salt that is not white, that has all the good trace minerals in it. It may be Celtic or Himalayan Salt from deep deposits in the earth that have all the preserved natural minerals. If you have white salt, it is not the right salt, it has been made to look good, but they removed all the minerals. Sources (of unprocessed sea salt) are available from health food stores.

15. Detoxify the Liver with Herbs and Nutrients (Nutritionist or Naturopath) Milk Thistle, Alpha Lipoic Acid, etc.

Number FIFTEEN, it is very important to help support the liver, the adrenals, and the rest of the body to detoxify. And you can do that with nutrients, such as Chlorella, and Cilantro, or you can do it with many different herbs including milk thistle; also other nutrients such as alpha-Lipoic acid are very helpful. These are also available from Life Extension, and Pure Encapsulations.

Note – the below is pulled from an article we wrote earlier – you can sign up for these free articles at http://thyroid-adrenal-solutions.com. This also applies to Step 16 on Heavy Metal Detox that follows.

The suggestion is made to start with a trial first to see how you respond. There is a caveat with some nutrients such as chlorella and cilantro. Some practitioners believe these substances can stir mercury up and cause it to redistribute in the tissues, so proceed cautiously whenever using such items. Do this especially if you have a number of silver (mercury) amalgam fillings. It is recommended you have any silver fillings removed safely by a holistic dentist trained in proper removal, and replaced with safe materials. Ask your dentist to see the material safety data sheet for the filling material, and Google the ingredients for safety reasons.

Finally, whatever you finally choose to detox with, start with a very low dosage every few hours on a regular schedule and see how you do. There are support groups on the internet who will coach you in proper detoxification. Dr. Andy Cutler, a research scientist has written an excellent book on detoxing mercury from the body if you care to Google him as a resource – some consider him to be a premier authority on such issues. Detoxification products are available from Life Extension, and Pure Encapsulations.

STEPS 16 – 20, HEAVY METAL DETOX, HERBS AND SUPPLEMENTS TO ELIMINATE YEAST, IODINE, VITAMIN D AND OTHER NEEDED VITAMINS AND MINERALS FOR THYROID AND ADRENALS

16. Heavy Metal Detox if Elevated Levels (May use oral DMSA, Zeolites, rectal EDTA suppositories, Chlorella, Cilantro)

We are at number SIXTEEN, Heavy Metal Detox. If you have elevated levels of metals, THEY can be measured with urinary tests through several companies, including Metametrix. But we find if they are elevated you need to do something to pull them out, to loosen them up, and to get rid of them. And this will help free up a lot of heavy metals that interfere with thyroid production. Mercury pretty much binds the enzyme that converts T4 to active T3, and paralyzes that enzyme. So it will dramatically help your thyroid if you can eliminate heavy metals out of your system. Some of the options may include oral DMSA, Zeolites, which are used as pills, sprays, and drops, there are even rectal EDTA Suppositories and other herbal sources like Chlorella and Cilantro can be very helpful.

17. Herbal, Supplements, Medications and Nutritional Consultation to Eliminate Yeast (Low Glycemic diet, many herbs etc)

Number SEVENTEEN is yeast. It is fairly common in many conditions, especially in low thyroid. There are many ways to eliminate yeast from the body. There are prescription medications and there are herbal medications. Absolutely you have to follow a low glycemic diet, minimize sugar, pop, and very high glycemic carbohydrates such as white bread, white flour, and white rice. The herbs that are helpful include oregano oil and Olive Leaf, and oftentimes reviewing your whole diet with a nutritionist will help stabilize and eliminate yeast from your body, because otherwise it creates havoc and many symptoms - achiness, sore joints, brain fog, and definitely digestive problems with gas, bloat, constipation, and diarrhea.

18. Iodine at 12.5 mg/day or more for Thyroid, Breast, Ovaries, Uterus and Prostate (typical intake healthy Japanese)

Number EIGHTEEN is Iodine which is critical for everybody, but absolutely essential if you have thyroid problems. Our bodies don't get enough from the salt that we eat. The problem is that Iodine is only added to the white salt that has been processed and all the minerals have been removed. So what you want to do is use only the unprocessed, natural sea salt that is usually pink or gray, this will have no iodine, and what you really need to do is mimic what the Japanese people do, and take iodine pills or eat sea vegetables, or take kelp tablets and try to get your iodine intake up to 10 or 12000 mg per day, which is the average for the Japanese, who live longer on this planet than any other nationality. They also have the lowest rate of breast cancer in any developed nation for their women. Iodine is what your thyroid uses to create thyroid hormones, either 3 or 4 iodine molecules, and all the other chemicals we are exposed to like bromine, fluoride, chlorine interfere and block this iodine we are getting, so we need to make sure we are getting adequate amounts to keep the thyroid functioning.

19. Vitamin D to keep 25 Hydroxy-D levels at 50-80 (50% Less Breast Cancer when Vitamin D levels over 52)

Number NINETEEN, Vitamin D is very important for health. It helps your thyroid; it lowers breast cancer risk, probably most cancer risks it lowers. It helps improve your immune system for flu, for infections, and it lowers the risk of diabetes, high blood pressure, and even multiple sclerosis. Your 25 Hydroxy vitamin D levels should be 50 to 80, and this is referenced per Dr. Hollick, who is a Vitamin D expert. Studies have shown that women have 50% less breast cancer when their vitamin D level is 52 or above. So it's very important to support your thyroid and your immune system by keeping your vitamin D levels adequate.

20. Add Vitamins and Minerals that are deficient (Doses depend on level of deficiency)

Number TWENTY is just to make sure that all the vitamins, minerals, nutrients that have been tested - that they are not deficient. Everything needs to work together in good working order, so your B Vitamins, your D, your Iodine, your Vitamin C, your amino acids, everything needs to be optimized for adequate and optimal functioning.

Steps 21 – 25, Adaptogenic Herbs, Saliva Testing for Adrenals, Food Allergy Panel, Probiotics and Nutrients for Gut Healing, and Natural Thyroid Hormone Therapy

21. Adaptogenic Herbs and Natural Hormones when needed (Ashwaganda, Ginseng, Rhodiola, Pregnenolone, DHEA, etc)

Number TWENTY ONE is adaptogenic herbs and natural hormones, and these are very helpful to support the thyroid. You need to make sure your DHEA and Pregnenolone are optimized. For any adrenal concerns, multiple adaptogenic herbs including Ashwaganda, Ginseng, and Rhodiola, etc. will help for energy and vitality. When your adrenals are functioning well that will help your thyroid.

22. Saliva Testing for Adrenals if any Fatigue, Exhaustion. Test saliva 4 times over 24 hours to evaluate your cycle

Number TWENTY TWO – Saliva Testing for Adrenals – if you have concerns and you're not sure, there are several companies including Diagnostics that will do a saliva test. Just do a little spit 4 times during the day and they can measure your DHEA and cortisol as it fluctuates through the daytime and evening. This is really much more accurate than one single blood test at one point in time. It will tell you if you are having adrenal fatigue or adrenal burnout, or high cortisol, maybe high stress; both of these may be detrimental to your thyroid function.

23. If any food allergens consider full food allergy panel from BioTek etc with 96 regular or vegetarian foods and spices

Number TWENTY THREE is for food allergies. If you have one or two of the common food allergens such as gluten or casein you may want to consider a whole panel, because often with leaky gut there may be other foods that have caused problems and you have become allergic to them. Several companies, including Bio-Tek will test 96 different food allergens by IGG from just several drops of blood that you can even do at home. Use a finger stick for blood and put it on a little card, dry it, and send it off. It is a fabulous way to get a very complete analysis, with minimal cost and time.

24. Probiotics and Nutrients for gut healing including Glutamine, Omega 3s, Aloe, MSM, Licorice, Colostrum

Number TWENTY FOUR; there are several nutrients that are very important for your gut healing and for inflammation. If you have food allergies or if you have yeast then you probably have leaky gut. Healing nutrients may include glutamine, the omega 3's, or Krill Oil, Aloe, MSM, licorice, and colostrum.

Coconut oil is good for gut health, good for thyroid, good for improving your weight, and may even have some benefits for brain health. So coconut oil is another simple, easy thing that you can add as a nutrient into your body.

Probiotics are essential for everyone, but certainly if there is gut inflammation, if you have food allergies, or if you have yeast. Again, probiotics mean you are putting the good bacteria in to replace the bad bacteria and yeast, and function of the intestines is dramatically improved and it even helps for weight loss and for mood problems and mental health.

25. Natural Thyroid Hormone Therapy as indicated, prescribed by a Physician, for men and for women

Last, number TWENTY FIVE, is utilizing natural thyroid hormone therapy like Armor or NatureThroid or West-Throid that your physician can order and can be obtained from a regular pharmacy; or compounded thyroid hormone from a compounding pharmacy. This can maximize the exact amount of T3 and T4 in your thyroid hormone pill by compounding it specifically for your needs. This is essential to make sure you have both T3 and T4 levels that are adequate.

Please note that prescribing of natural thyroid hormone is the last step; there is a chance that by following all the previous steps in order that you may not need this medication. Perhaps adding in some natural foods or supplements and eliminating toxins will have you feeling top notch with no need for anything else. A natural remedy of the situation is always best, but many do find natural thyroid hormone to be helpful.

Conclusion

In summary, we covered a number of topics including proper thyroid and adrenal testing, thyroid and adrenal toxins to avoid, as well as helpful supplements for thyroid and adrenals, critical nutrients, including iodine for thyroid and adrenal performance, and natural thyroid hormone therapy that, if needed, will help your thyroid's performance. The emphasis was on natural, alternative health therapies and solutions; solutions that would help you feel your best, lose weight, and have more energy, letting you live a less stressful life.

The benefits you gained from this e-book are hopefully many. If you proceeded through this book step-by-step, you will first know if your thyroid is afflicted, and then know how to treat it, what toxins to avoid, helpful thyroid and adrenal supplements to take, what level of iodine to take, and nutrients that can help you feel better, heal your gut, and boost your metabolism, including thyroid.

By buying certain food items, and being selective when purchasing food for your family, you can really improve the quality of what you eat. In addition, growing your own garden, and buying from local organic farmers who do not use pesticides is a great idea.

Another major benefit from application of what you learned is if your thyroid has been an obstacle to weight loss. Perhaps it may not be any longer with the steps you have taken and you may shed unnecessary pounds. But whether you need to lose weight or not, having thyroid and adrenals that are in top notch condition will benefit you for life.

Thank you for joining us!

Diane Culik MD

ABC Wellness

Did You Like This Book?

Let everyone know by posting a review on Amazon.

Just click here and it will take you directly to the reviews page:

What to do now: Don't miss out on a free thyroid video, and tons of free articles, gifts, eBooks from ABC Wellness and more! Please visit us at the website listed below:

(To see a free video and for an even more comprehensive video based program,

please visit **http://thyroid-adrenal-solutions.com**)

Other Books by ABC Wellness in the "Simple Steps to Better Health" Series:

Calming Inflammation: The eBook "<u>Autoimmune and Inflammation Solutions</u>" gives you a Natural Recovery Protocol to Overcome Food Allergies, Gluten, GMOs, EMFs, Biofilms, Yeast or Candida Overgrowth. Only 99 cents!

Dental and Heart Care: The eBook, "<u>Reversing Gum And Heart Disease</u>" provides a Protocol to Lower hs-CRP, and Heal Inflammation Through a Paleo Diet, Dental Care, and Targeted Nutrients and Supplements. Only $2.99!

Thyroid and Adrenal Facts: The eBook "<u>Thyroid Adrenal Secrets Revealed</u>" teaches you what you the 10 top things you need to know before you see your doctor for thyroid or adrenal issues.

Analyze and Improve Your Health: The eBook "<u>25 Step Healing Program</u>" gives you simple steps to take to evaluate your health and improve it by correcting deficiencies.

Improve Your Health Safely: The eBook "<u>Heal Your Whole Body Naturally</u>" covers using bio identical hormones as well as a natural approach to staying well.

Lose Pounds Quickly by Overcoming Obstacles to Weightloss: The eBook "<u>The ABC Wellness</u>

Weightloss Pyramid" covers 9 major obstacles or possible roadblocks that once removed will help you lose weight without dieting or exercise, though that is recommended to compound your gains.

Acid Reflux or GERD: The eBook "Acid Reflux Relief Now" allows you to stop heartburn or acid reflux in its tracks with natural remedies.

Anti-Aging Secrets: The eBook "Insider Bio Identical Hormone Secrets and More" covers the secrets you need to know to stay young and health with the use of natural hormones.

Longevity and Anti-Aging Advice: The eBook "How to Live to 100 – Top Dos and Don'ts" gives you the top 10 dos and don'ts you should follow if you want to reach and surpass the golden age of 100.

Thyroid, Adrenals and Weightloss: The eBook "Thyroid Adrenal Weightloss Solutions" covers the 25 steps in the "25 Step Healing Program" book, along with more information on losing pounds quickly.

Special note on Thyroid Adrenal Weightloss Solutions: This is a modified version of the "25 Step Healing Program" eBook, so please purchase this one if you want more information on losing weight as well as the thyroid, adrenal and testing information.

ABC Wellness "Simple Steps to Better Health!"

Please forgive us if any sites referenced in our eBooks are not operational when you visit them, and please try back later, as they may be under construction. Thank-you!

Special Announcements

To see a free video on thyroid adrenal care and for an even more comprehensive video based program, and for free gifts and articles on thyroid and adrenals by email, please visit and sign up at http://thyroid-adrenal-solutions.com

www.ingramcontent.com/pod-product-compliance
Lightning Source LLC
Chambersburg PA
CBHW071352280526
45787CB00001B/293